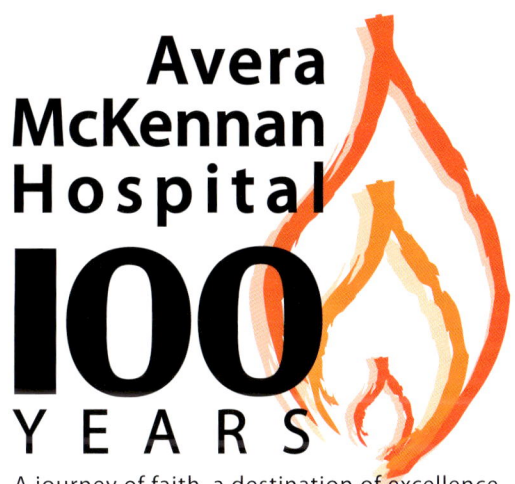

Avera
McKennan
Hospital
100
YEARS

A journey of faith, a destination of excellence

Published by The Donning Company Publishers
184 Business Park Drive, Suite 206, Virginia Beach, VA 23462

Library of Congress Cataloging-in-Publication Data

Preston, Margaret H. (Margaret Helen)
  A journey of faith, a destination of excellence : Avera McKennan
Hospital's first century of caring / Margaret Preston.
       p. ; cm.
  Includes bibliographical references and index.
  ISBN 978-1-57864-660-9 (hard cover : alk. paper) -- ISBN 978-1-57864-661-6
(soft cover : alk. paper)
  1. Avera McKennan Hospital & University Health Center--History. 2.
Hospitals--South Dakota--Sioux Falls--History. 3. Catholic hospitals--South
Dakota--Sioux Falls--History. 4. Academic medical centers--South
Dakota--Sioux Falls--History. I. Title.
  [DNLM: 1. Avera McKennan Hospital & University Health Center. 2.
Hospitals, Religious--history--South Dakota. 3. History, 20th
Century--South Dakota. 4. Missions and Missionaries--history--South Dakota.
WX 28 AS8]
  RA982.S5652A94 2010
  362.1109783'371--dc22
                            2010045774

A Journey of Faith,
A Destination of Excellence:

Avera McKennan Hospital's
First Century of Caring

Margaret Preston, Ph.D.

With all good wishes

Margaret Preston

Dedication

This book is dedicated to the Presentation and Benedictine Sisters and to the
thousands of physicians and employees past, present and future whose dedication
and care sustain the Avera McKennan ministry of healing.

A Journey of Faith,
A Destination of Excellence:
Avera McKennan Hospital's
First Century of Caring

Acknowledgements

The legacy of this work is not the written pages that provide only the most abbreviated history of Avera McKennan Hospital & University Health Center but it is the many interviews with current and former employees that supply the true story. Most were done by Ms. Kathleen McGreevy, the former director of communications for Avera Health and editor of the system's internal newspaper called *All of Us*. To date, McGreevy has left an archive of some 14 volumes with over 50 interviews of persons connected with the hospital. And the process continues. These interviews offer insight into the nature of the hospital and the importance of its mission. What comes through in almost all of the interviews is that the Sisters who run this hospital have ensured that the healing ministry of Jesus, as espoused in the Avera mission statement, is maintained. This mission, in its broadest sense, appears to have permeated throughout the organization—the result of the hard work of the Sisters who, in spite of decreased numbers, continue to be a presence in the hospital and throughout the Avera Health system.

The writing of this history is the result of serendipitous meetings that not only put me in touch with Ms. Kathleen McGreevy but with most of her family as well. Avera McKennan owes Ms. McGreevy a debt of gratitude for having the foresight to recognize the importance of interviewing persons affiliated with the hospital—including some who have since passed away. The many persons who sat for interviews and spoke of their own history with McKennan Hospital must be thanked as their words will be held in posterity for the 200th anniversary.

I would like to thank Ms. Donna Farris, writer/editor for Avera McKennan, whose writing and editorial work has greatly improved this manuscript. Thanks must be offered to the unnamed persons who kept the scrapbooks in which articles, letters and in-house news are contained. Sr. Lois Ann Sargent, archivist of the Presentation Convent in Aberdeen has been a supportive resource and a wonderful host. The women of the Aberdeen convent are welcoming to the stranger and always excited to learn the plans of the researcher. Ms. Janice Nims, the Rev. Kathryn Timpany and the Rev. Ryan Otto of First Congregational Church in Sioux Falls were most helpful and always excited to hear that a former member as prominent as Helen McKennan would be getting further recognition. Thanks must be offered to the staff of the Old Courthouse Museum and particularly Mr. Kevin Gansz, curator of education. The librarians at the downtown Siouxland Library were ever patient as I trolled through years of the *Argus Leader* on microfilm. The librarians of the Swan Library in Albion, New York must be thanked for their efforts to track down evidence on Helen and William McKennan. My colleagues at Augustana College, and particularly the staff of the Mikkelsen Library, have helped, listened and supported me during this process.

The friends I now have at Avera McKennan, particularly in the Marketing Department, are many and I thank them. Ms. Jessica Potter must be recognized for her beautiful design work that brings this history to life. I must particularly acknowledge Mr. Russell McKnight whom, in addition to his insightful advice on writing this history, has become a good friend. Thanks must be extended to Sr. Mary Thomas, Sr. Colman Coakley and the other Sisters who read this manuscript. Others who have read various versions of this manuscript must also be acknowledged and these include Dr. Julia Bennet, Ms. LaVonne Gaspar, Ms. Michelle Lavallee, Ms. Kathleen McGreevy, Mr. Richard Molseed, Dr. Margaret Ó hÓgartaigh, Dr. Robert Preston, Ms. Robin Prunty, Mr. Fred Slunecka and Mr. Jim Ward. The years of this project included the birth of my beautiful daughter Frances who, along with Nick, Greg and my husband Rick Lundberg, I thank for their love and patience throughout this long process.

This project has been supported by grants from the South Dakota Humanities Council, Avera McKennan, the Augustana College Research and Scholarly Activities Committee and the Cushwa Center for the Study of American Catholicism, University of Notre Dame.

Introduction

*Avera is a health ministry rooted in the Gospel.
Our mission is to make a positive impact
in the lives and health of persons and communities
by providing quality services
guided by Christian values.*

Every year since 2006 Avera McKennan Hospital & University Health Center has been named one of the 100 Top Hospitals® in the nation by Thomson Reuters. This is only one of the many awards the hospital has received over its 100-year history and the earning of so many accolades is certainly a testament to the hospital's many physicians and employees. No institutional history can include the names of everyone, both past and present, who have worked to make it a success. This story is only able to include some of the people and some of the departments within Avera McKennan, but this in no way diminishes the contributions made by all.

During the last 100 years, Avera McKennan has seen both good times and bad. Yet, even during the tougher stretches the hospital has sought to always maintain its mission, recognizing that failure to adhere to its guiding principles will set any organization adrift. The Sisters of the Presentation of the Blessed Virgin Mary have led the hospital from its inception and it is they, now joined by the Benedictine Sisters, who continue to ensure that Avera Health is the largest Catholic medical system on America's northern plains.

Since the hospital's dedication on December 17, 1911, the people of Sioux Falls have always offered their support and Avera McKennan is most grateful to them. From the hospital's earliest days, when the community provided us with linens to the present when annually over 1,000 volunteers donate their time, Avera McKennan has been thankful for the generosity of the local community. We hope that this goodwill can forever continue.

Avera McKennan looks forward to a very bright future. Through the recognition of its interesting past, we can see how this hospital has become an integral part of the future of Sioux Falls, the state of South Dakota and beyond. While every name cannot be acknowledged, this centennial history seeks to express its appreciation to the many persons who have sought to sustain the mission of Avera McKennan and participate in the healing ministry of Jesus.

Fred Slunecka
Avera Health Chief Operating Officer

Sr. Mary Thomas
Avera McKennan Senior Vice President for Mission Services

On January 28, 1911 the *Argus Leader* announced:

"SIOUX FALLS'

MAGNIFICENT NEW HOSPITAL UNDER CONSTRUCTION."

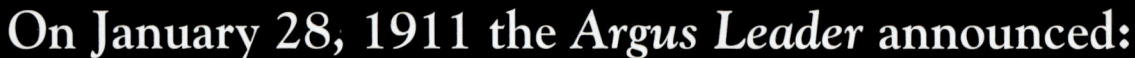

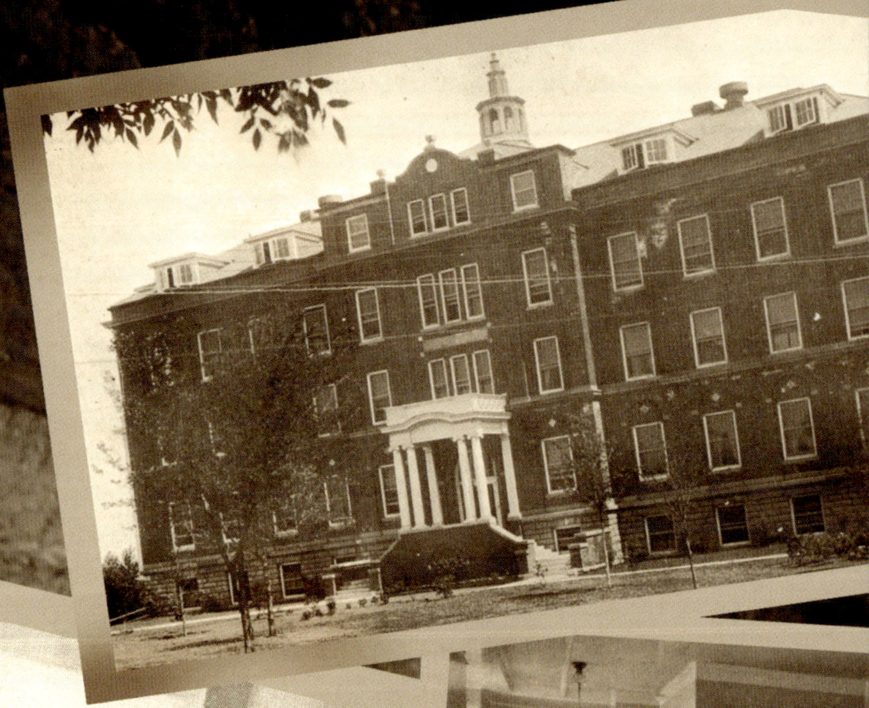

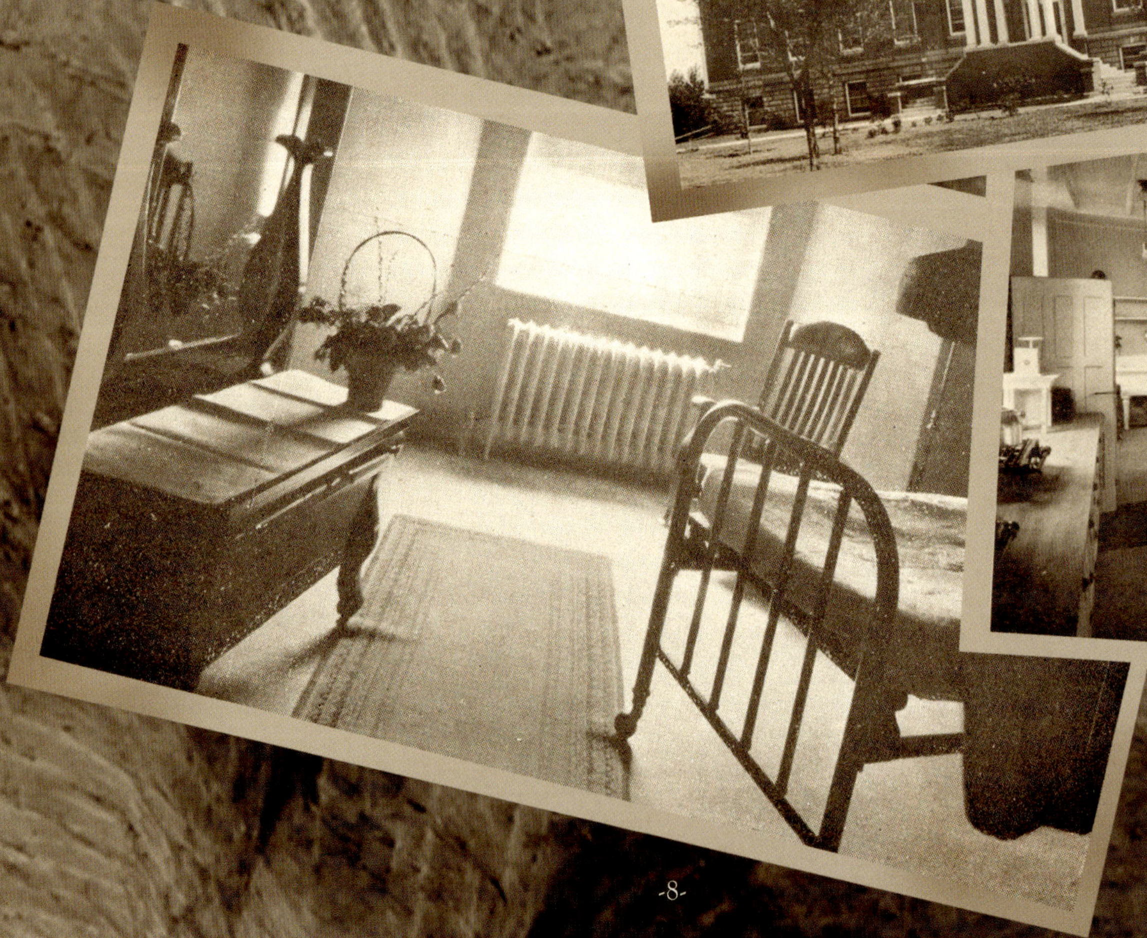

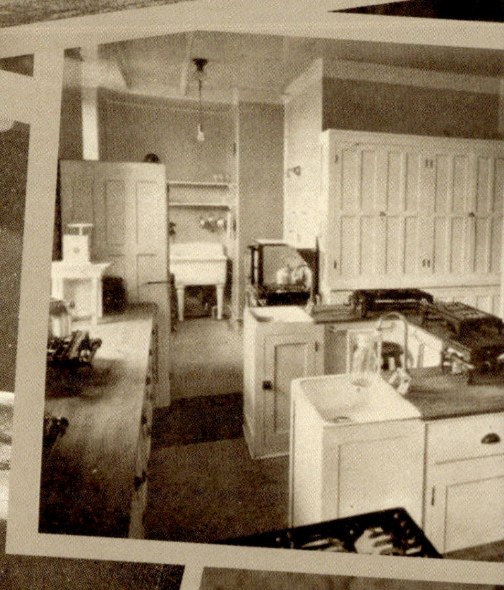

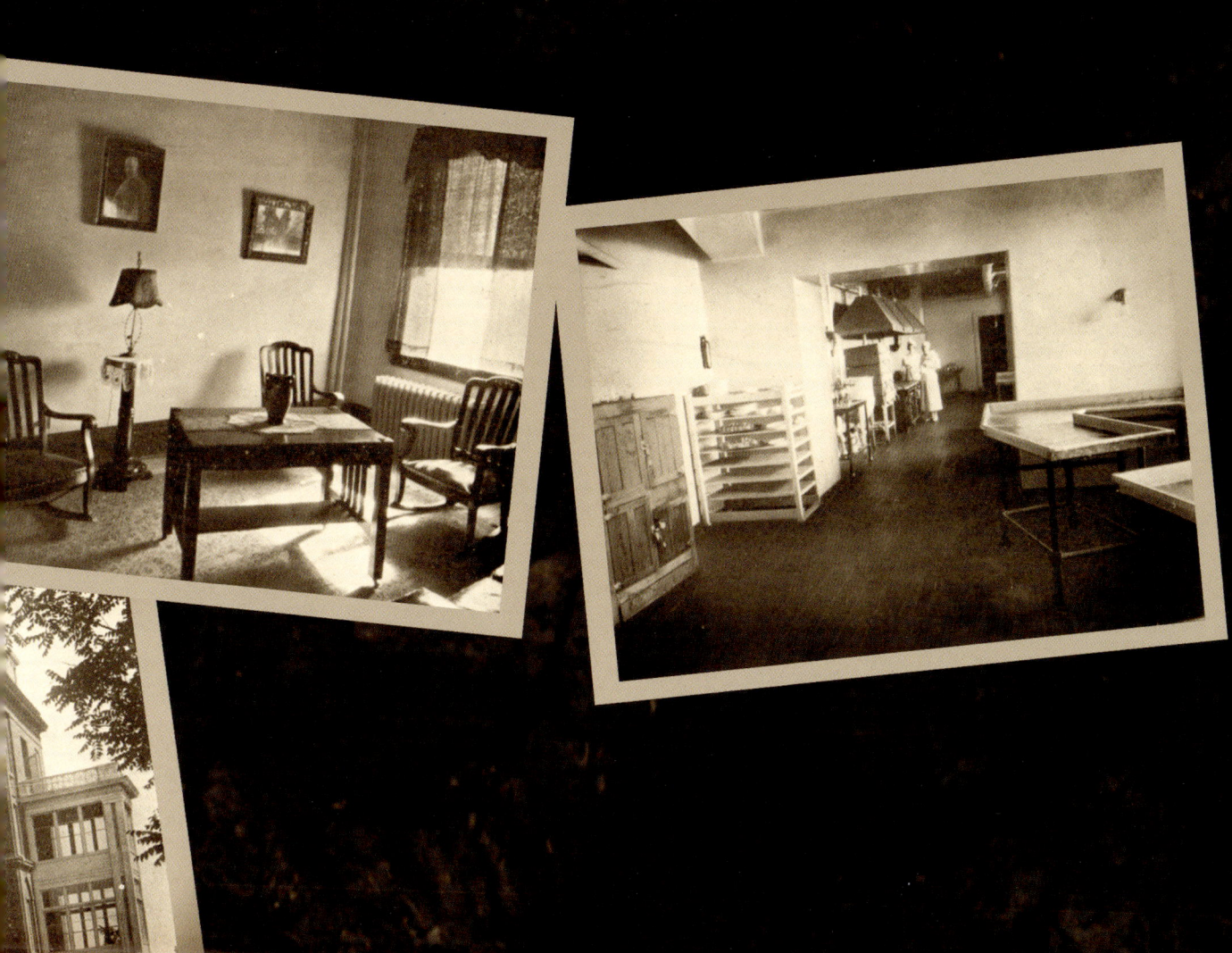

The article discussed local anticipation that, as the temperatures in Sioux Falls slowly warmed, construction would resume on a gift to the city—a new hospital. It would be named for Helen McKennan; the woman who willed the seed money for a hospital. The paper noted that "the building will also be absolutely fire proof and as sanitary as modern ingenuity will make it." The article went on to discuss that the second and third floors would offer over 30 private rooms with over half of these with private baths while the fourth floor would house a small operating room and "a large surgeons and consulting room" as well as 16 more private rooms. The fifth story, or attic, would also have private rooms and a community room. Finally, many hospitals at that time provided housing for nursing students and McKennan offered its nurses accommodation that included sitting rooms near their private bedrooms.[1]

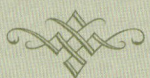

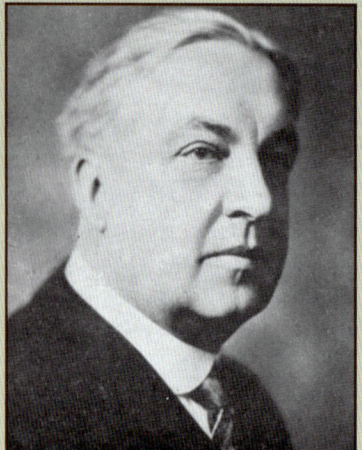

Dr. Edwin L. Perkins

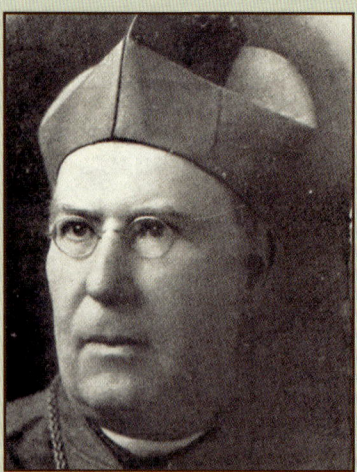

Bishop Thomas O'Gorman

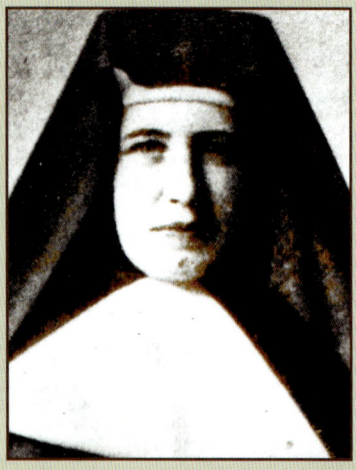

Mother Joseph Butler

The *Argus Leader* described the modern amenities as including electricity throughout, telephone service, elevator and dumb waiter. The 'silent signal' service, which was lights instead of ringing bells, prevented any noise that might be annoying to patients. All of this provided Sioux Falls, as the paper noted, with an institution that "will compare with [those in] even larger cities." The newspaper updated readers again in June as the slate roof was completed and plumbing installed; the paper predicted that the hospital would be ready by October. It noted, however, that the costs were inching higher, surpassing the expected $60,000 and edging toward $90,000—possibly the result of an added underground tunnel that connected the boiler and laundry rooms with the hospital.

Eventually, trustees of McKennan's will sought a loan for the extra money and also "borrowed the legacy, which totaled $27,742.54, from the Helen McKennan Hospital Fund, and thus started a perpetual return of interest to the fund." This would then continue to draw annual interest and, as Helen McKennan desired, be used to pay hospital expenses for worthy, needy patients.[2] Ultimately, the hospital cost $110,000 to build.[3] Finally, the *Argus Leader* emphasized that "while the local hospital is not as large as many, it can safely be said that there is not a more up-to-date and better equipped hospital in the northwest."[4] The trustees of McKennan's will already had determined who would administer the hospital. In 1910, Dr. Edwin L. Perkins, Helen McKennan's personal physician and a trustee of her will, approached Dr. T.J. Billion and asked if he would speak about the idea of a hospital with his good friend and Sioux Falls Roman Catholic Bishop, Thomas O'Gorman.[5] O'Gorman then wrote to Mother Joseph Butler, Superior of the Sisters of the Presentation of the Blessed Virgin Mary, or Presentation Sisters.[6] By that time, the Presentation Order already ran hospitals in Aberdeen and Mitchell and, despite the fact that the Sisters were in the process of opening a third hospital in Miles City, Mont., Mother Joseph consented to operate a fourth hospital in Sioux Falls.

O'Gorman said that the name of the hospital had been left up to him and he had "no hesitation calling it the McKennan Hospital in honor of and gratitude to the noble-hearted woman" who left a legacy for the establishment of the hospital. O'Gorman made clear that the hospital would be a place where patients of all faiths and ministers of those faiths would be welcomed and that in the hospital, the doctors of the body and the doctors of the soul "will find here the perfect democracy of Christianity." O'Gorman then dedicated the building to the glory of God and blessed all who would work in it or need its care in the memory of a "noble woman."

The dedication was set for Sunday, December 17, 1911.[7] There was limited space for a public gathering and thus the trustees issued personal invitations to such persons as ministers of the gospel, doctors, dentists, nurses and city officers among others. Later, the public would be invited to tour the hospital.

At 4 p.m. on December 17 "with impressive ceremonies" and in the presence of 200 attendees, the hospital was dedicated. A number of local dignitaries spoke at the ceremony, including Bishop O'Gorman and E.A. Sherman, executor of Helen McKennan's will.[8]

In his opening remarks, O'Gorman first reflected on Helen McKennan's bequest noting that it was not only visionary but, he hoped, inspirational:

"Yonder is McKennan Park intended to prevent disease, here is McKennan Hospital intended to cure or relieve disease. Are not these institutions a fit tribute to a noble Christian woman? May they prove to be an inspiration of philanthropic benevolence to many other citizens of Sioux Falls."[9]

E.A. Sherman, Helen McKennan's good friend, continued with this theme by reminding the attendees that as her illness caused McKennan to increasingly struggle during her last months, she came to feel that she wanted to use her wealth to serve humanity. Sherman said that McKennan knew that after she left some money to her church, close friends and family, what remained would not be enough "to found and maintain, independently of other funds, any public institution." Yet, she resisted giving the funds to various charities because this would not "centralize and accomplish what she had in mind." Sherman stated that McKennan wanted to aid the indigent sick thus she was determined to form a trust to control and fulfill her dream. Sherman concluded by stating that he was satisfied that Helen McKennan, so far as she was able, left the money that "forms the cornerstone" of the institution "which stands on this commanding elevation, overlooking the park grounds provided by her generous impulse for the pleasure and benefit of the people."[10]

As the dedication ceremony proceeded, the hospital staff was preparing for its first patient. A call came to the hospital for Dr. Gilbert Cottam, McKennan's Chief of Staff, from Dr. H.F. Moore of Worthington, Minn., who stated that he was going to drive a man to Sioux Falls for an emergency appendectomy. The hospital was not meant to open its doors for another two weeks, and Sister Rose McCormick recalled that she felt the hospital was not yet ready to have a patient. Nevertheless, the surgery had to await the completion of the dedication services, as well as the retrieval of surgical tools.[11] At 11 p.m., some seven hours after the McKennan Hospital dedication, Dr. Cottam operated on a man from Beresford, S.D. Years later, Dr. Cottam's son, Dr. Geoffrey Cottam, wrote Sister Colman Coakley about his father's surgery and noted that Bishop O'Gorman was invited to witness the procedure…which apparently he did![12]

This successful appendectomy was quickly followed the next day by a second emergency appendectomy on a man from Rock Rapids, Iowa, while two additional patients appeared that same day.[13] It is not a surprise

that local doctors wanted to get their patients into a hospital that was clearly equipped with the latest technology. While doctors had been performing appendectomies since the 18th century and had "perfected" the procedure by the 19th, the hospital was a much more sanitary environment and, in the hospital, Cottam had easy access to ether which had been used in surgery since 1846.[14]

Patients kept coming and McKennan Hospital welcomed its first infant just 10 days after the dedication when a boy was born to a Sioux Falls couple.[15] Within weeks of the dedication, McKennan Hospital was officially incorporated. Mother Joseph Butler would be the board of trustee's vice president while Sister Agatha Collins would act as the board's treasurer as well as the hospital's first superior administrator.[16] In addition, the three trustees (discussed below) that Helen McKennan had designated to be responsible for ensuring the hospital's establishment were to continue to be involved with the hospital. Thus, Colonel Thomas H. Brown was president and Dr. Edwin Perkins secretary of the board of trustees while Mr. John Mallanney would act as secretary of the Helen G. McKennan fund.[17] While the hospital was certainly on its way, there was still much that the institution needed and the community offered its support.

A few months after the hospital opened, the "women of Sioux Falls" welcomed McKennan to the community by hosting a linen shower planned by a committee which canvassed Sioux Falls for donations of anything…even one towel, pillowslip or sheet. "The result has been an overwhelming success" announced the *Argus Leader* and among the donations were enough curtains to cover all of the hospital's windows. Mother Joseph was in attendance during the reception on the afternoon of February 15, and she welcomed "hundreds of women" who came to visit the hospital and "show their interest in the new institution." The *Argus Leader* noted that the success of the event showed the good feeling of cooperation between the "good women" of Sioux Falls and the hospital; a budding relationship "which will prove to be of great advantage to the institution in the passing years."[18]

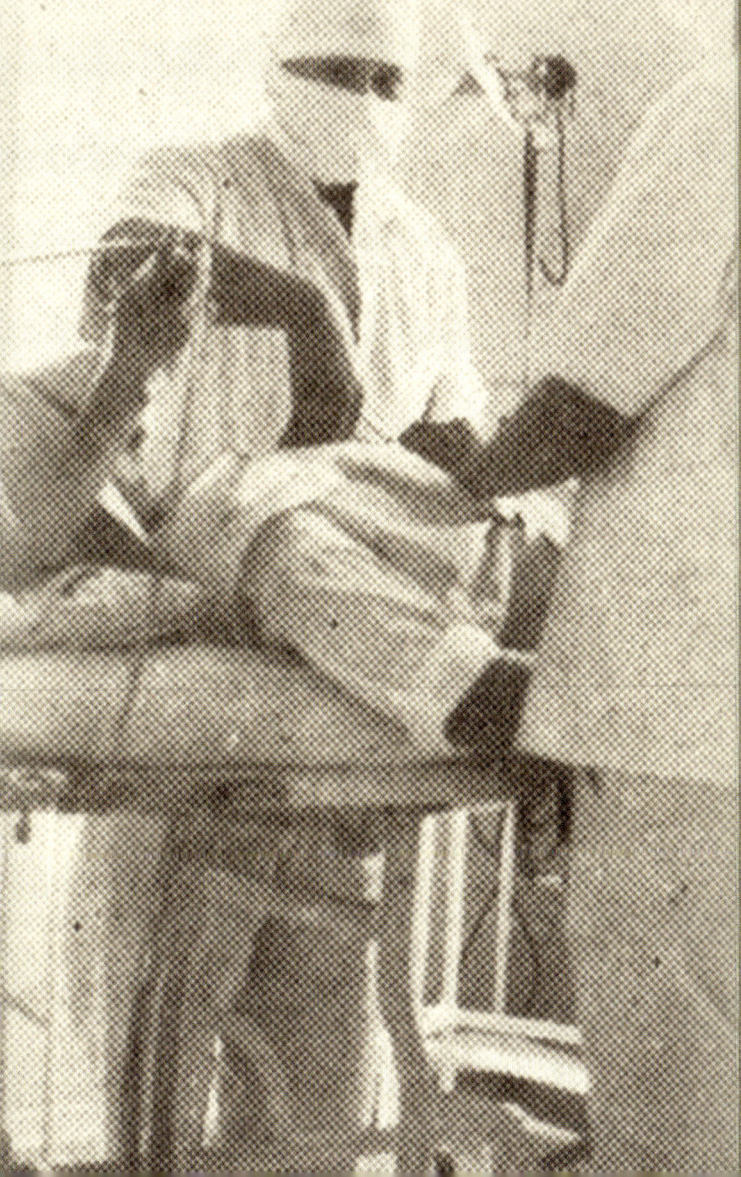

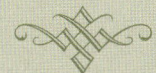

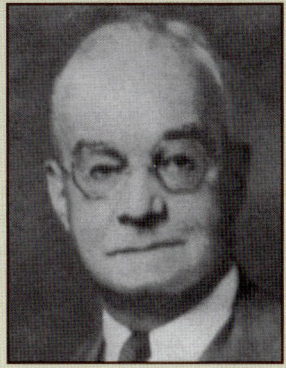

Dr. Gilbert Cottam

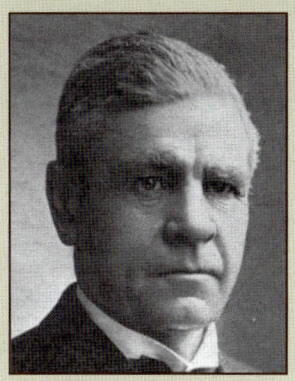

Colonel
Thomas H. Brown

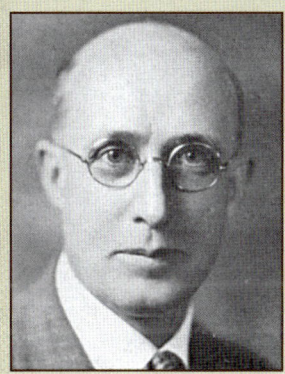

Dr. T.J. Billion

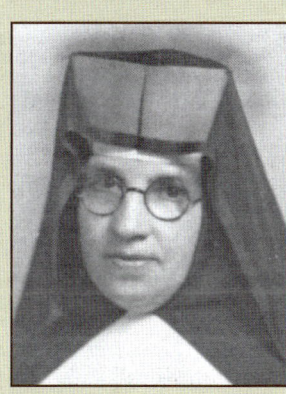

Sister Agatha Collins

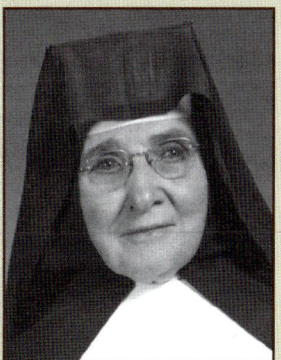

Sister Rose McCormick

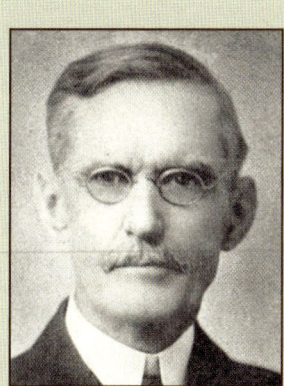

John Mallanney

HELEN MCKENNAN (1841-1906)
a "woman of broad education and wide sympathies"

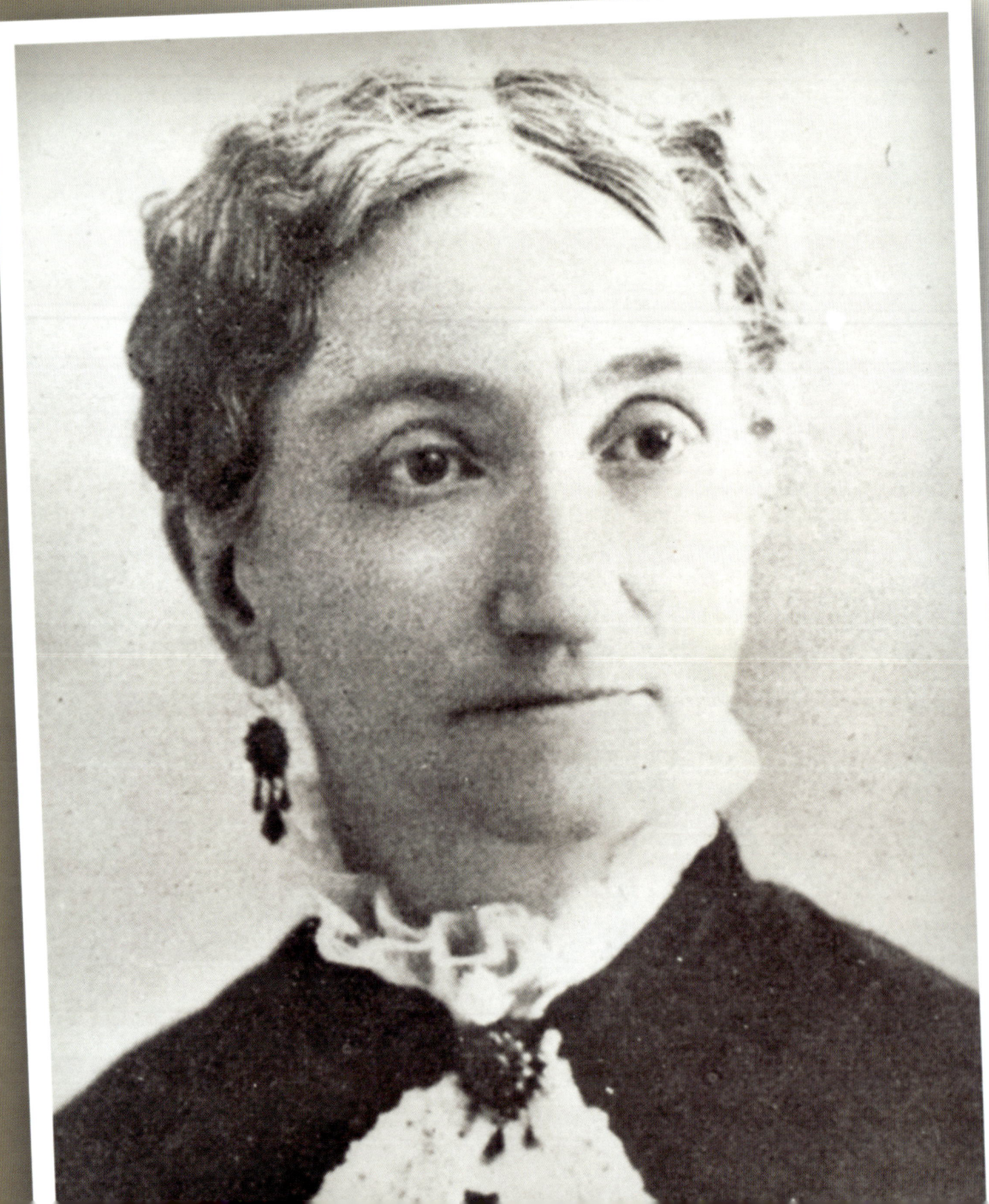

"A Good Woman Gone":
Helen McKennan

When Helen McKennan looked out of the window of her
Sioux Falls mansion, she saw the 80 acres that surrounded
her home, a scene that Edwin A. Sherman, father of the
Sioux Falls parks system, described as "unsurpassed."[19] While
McKennan was certainly the granddame of early 20th century
Sioux Falls, she could also be described as a representative
of the late Victorian era: a philanthropist who sought to
help those in greatest need. The long 19th century, which
historians often do not end until World War I, saw the rise
of the woman philanthropist. These were women who,
because their middle or upper-class status restricted them
from respectably engaging in a paid profession, instead were
active in charitable causes. In many ways it was these women,
and religious orders of women included, who helped lay the
foundation for the Western World's modern social service
system. Helen McKennan was just such a woman.

A member of the Sioux Falls Congregational Church,

... Helen McKennan left most of her worldly possessions to Sioux Falls.

Little is known about Helen Gale McKennan and what we
do know generally comes from the evidence of her generosity.
Helen Gale was born in Albion, N.Y., on September 6, 1841,
to Elizabeth Decker and David Gale. Helen was from a large
family; the 1855 census for Orleans County lists Helen's
mother, by then a widow, as residing in a home with,

in addition to Helen, daughters Phoebe, Margaret and Frances as well as a son, Gabriel.* Not listed was Helen's brother Artemus who, in 1854, moved to St. Paul where he engaged in a grain and mercantile business.[20]

Helen was described as a "woman of broad education and wide sympathies" having traveled throughout the United States and beyond. She spent a short time in Sioux Falls in 1874 visiting her brother Artemus, but returned to Albion to marry physician William McKennan. McKennan, born in Herkimer, N.Y., in July of 1817, he entered the College of Physicians and Surgeons, now Columbia University, and graduated in 1847. After briefly practicing in Middleport, N.Y., McKennan moved to Albion in 1852 and married Miss Harriet Guild, a local school teacher. Harriet died on June 2, 1872.

William McKennan spent the rest of his life in Albion, where he "attained a high eminence in the practice of medicine." A founding member of the Orleans County Medical Society in 1873, McKennan was clearly well respected by his colleagues. After she returned to Albion in 1874, Helen Gale married William McKennan; sadly, the union was brief as Dr. McKennan died at the age of 62 on August 21, 1879, leaving behind Helen, then 38.[21]

In the early 1890s, Helen McKennan returned to Sioux Falls to work with her brother, Artemus, a member of the Dakota Land Company. Artemus Gale, who was 16 years older than Helen, had also been a successful real estate agent in St. Paul. He moved to Sioux Falls after 1870, where he added to his real-estate holdings and was a charter member of First Congregational Church.[22] It appears that Helen McKennan was a partner in her brother's real estate dealings, owning half interest in the 80 acres that surrounded her Sioux Falls home as well as "a section of farmland in Lincoln County and numerous lots within the city."[23]

"A Good Woman Gone" read the *Argus Leader*'s headline as it described the funeral of Helen McKennan on October 2, 1906. In addition to the many Sioux Falls residents who came to pay their respects, Mayor Pillsbury, in recognition of her contributions to the city, sent a contingent of six aldermen and six city councilors to attend the funeral. The Rev. Frank Fox, pastor of First Congregational Church, presided and spoke of how McKennan hoped to live on so as to help her brother Artemus, but knew that her "malady would prove fatal." The Rev. Fox described McKennan as having lived a full life which included a grand tour of Europe and travel to the Orient where she "visited the homes of the missionaries and knew well their modes of living and their problems of life."

In her will, McKennan left First Congregational Church $500 and a quarter section of land. The church sold the land for $5,000 and used the money to buy a site and build a new church.[24] Fox next described how McKennan left all that she had to others. To begin, she left 20 acres for a park and stated that she sought to ensure that the park was "a place where mothers and their children can come and enjoy the fresh air, the sunshine, and the cooling shade. I want it to be a place of rest where the Sabbath may be respected."[25]

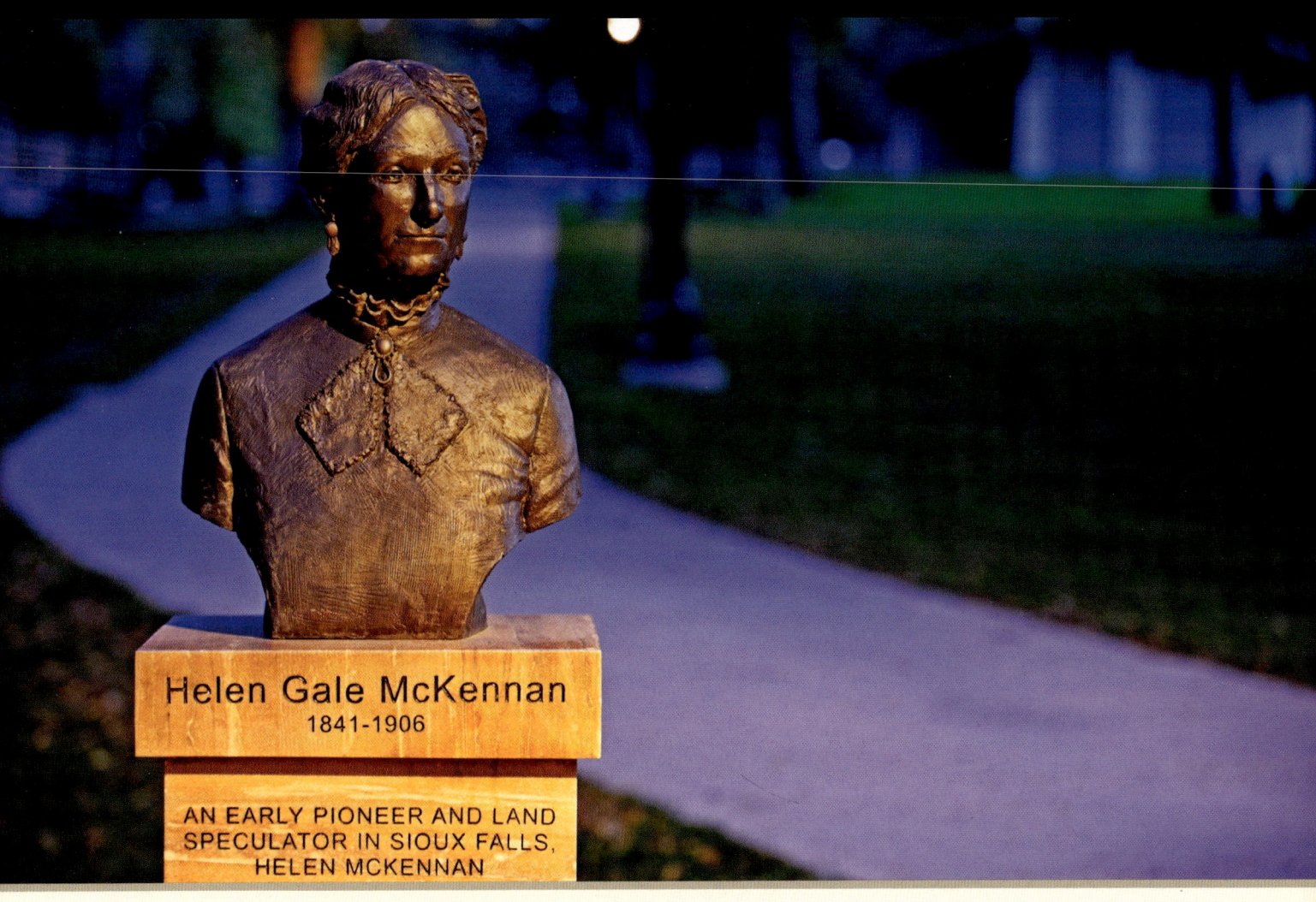

Helen Gale McKennan
1841-1906

AN EARLY PIONEER AND LAND
SPECULATOR IN SIOUX FALLS,
HELEN MCKENNAN

Fox went on to challenge those who questioned McKennan's decision to give away her worldly possessions, noting that they would eventually "understand her eternal worth" and that what she had done "shall be spoken of for a memorial of her."[26]

As Fox pointed out, the park was not McKennan's only gift to Sioux Falls. Fully half of Helen McKennan's estate went toward the "betterment" of the city.[27] McKennan sought to put some of the money toward an institution that would provide medical care to Sioux Falls' neediest citizens. Coincidentally, on August 20, 1906—just a month before McKennan's death, the *Argus Leader* published an article titled "Need a Hospital" in which Yankton physician Dr. V. Sebaikin-Ross told a reporter that Sioux Falls was in "the great need of an up-to-date hospital."[28]

Interestingly, according to Sherman, Helen McKennan made her decision to dedicate money toward a hospital in the last few weeks of her life. Little could Dr. Sebaikin-Ross have guessed that Helen McKennan had provided in her will that $25,000 be used to establish another hospital in Sioux Falls.

McKennan designated three trustees to find an organization to establish the hospital: Dr. Edwin L. Perkins, Col. Thomas H. Brown and Mr. John Mallanney*. They oversaw the sale of some of her property, with the resulting funds "applied by them toward constructing and furnishing a free public hospital in the city of Sioux Falls," as the *Argus Leader* reported. Dr. Perkins was Helen McKennan's private physician. They probably first met at First Congregational, where both were members.

Colonel Brown arrived in Sioux Falls in 1872 and, with his wife Mary Morse, was involved in the early development of the city and sought to bring improvements to Sioux Falls by spearheading, among other things, paving and lighting throughout the city. McKennan may have met Brown through her brother, who also arrived in Sioux Falls in the early 1870s and the two likely moved in the same business circles. In 1889, Colonel Brown became a partner in Brown and Saenger, which sells business products (and still bears his name). The third trustee, John Mallanney, worked for North Western Life Insurance Company, but little is known of him or how he met Helen McKennan.[29]

By the time Helen McKennan had returned to Sioux Falls in the early 1890s, the city was a much different place than it had been just a few decades earlier. Sioux Falls had become a metropolis of over 10,000, and rail transport was turning it into a market town. Other enhancements to the city included improvement in public lighting, sewer systems and organized police and fire protection. McKennan was likely aware of increasing efforts by urban planners throughout the United States to improve the health of city dwellers by supplying clean drinking water, better waste removal

and even the creation of urban parks and recreational areas.[30] Already Helen McKennan might have known that by 1900, Chicago, Kansas City and Buffalo, to name a few, had begun "multipurpose park systems."[31] Thus, McKennan's insightful gift of a park that offered, she hoped, "tired mothers" a place to seek "rest and health," also added Sioux Falls to this list of more progressive places.[32]

In addition to growing expectations for improved municipal services, cities found themselves also seeking to develop facilities that offered their citizens medical care. As settlers came west after the Homestead Act of 1862, with them traveled doctors who, in addition to wanting their own land, sought to differentiate themselves from the many physicians who populated America's growing East Coast cities. What these doctors found was a place where their reputation and prosperity could rise or fall on being quick-witted and resourceful.[33] Many of these physicians spent much of their time trying to convince residents of the benefits of various sanitary practices, including the proper disposal of waste as well as the importance of clean water. As immigrants settled the prairies, doctors first used horse and buggy and then cars to make house calls

Sioux Falls Lutheran Hospital

Moe Hospital

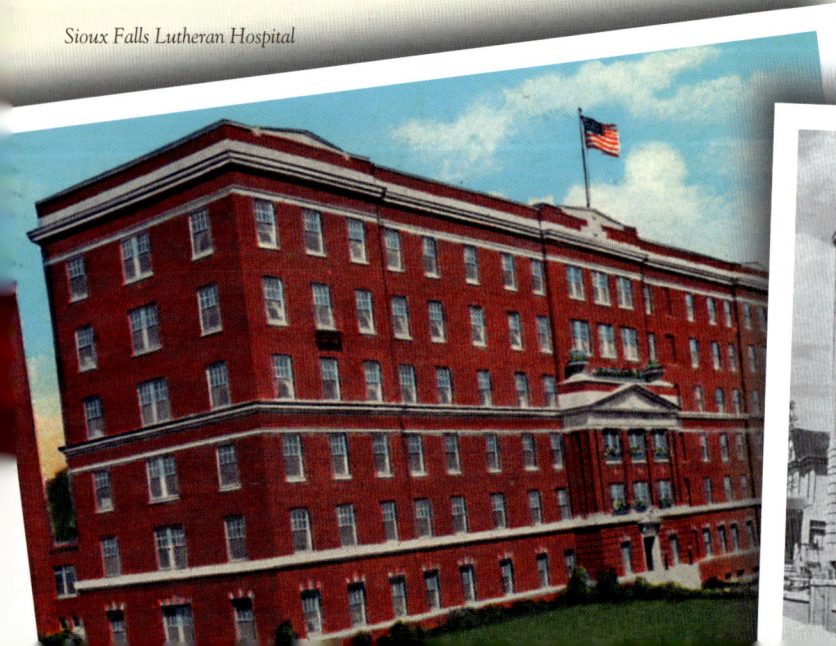

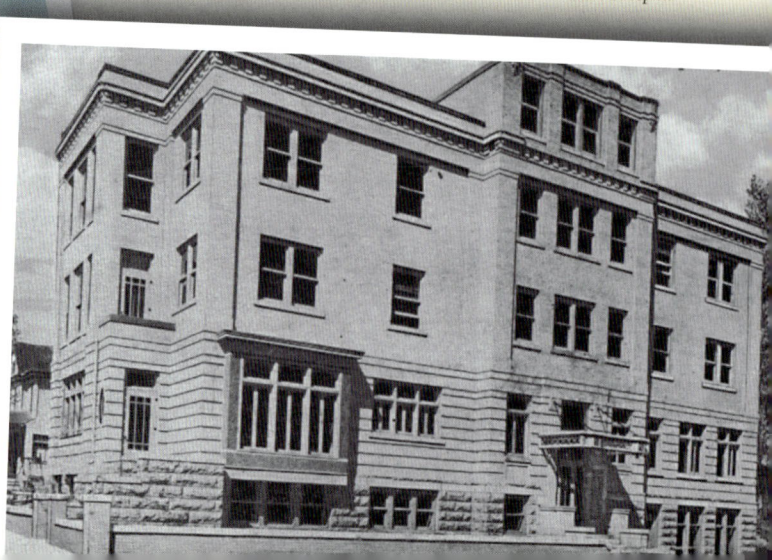

but, increasingly, they sent their most challenging cases to hospitals. Hospitals of the late 18th and early 19th century had been seen as places to which those who could not afford a house call went. Yet with improved medical technology, enhanced understanding of sterilization and growing knowledge of germ theory and vaccination, the hospital increasingly became an acceptable site for health care.[34]

In Sioux Falls, in 1894, a group of businessmen, clergy and doctors met to discuss the creation of a hospital for the city—the future Sioux Valley Hospital. First opened in a house located near Terrace Park, the hospital continued to grow and plans to build a new structure were discussed; in 1900, the hospital's directors purchased land near 19th Street and Minnesota avenue.[35] Construction began immediately, and that year Sioux Falls Lutheran Hospital, South Dakota's first community hospital, opened.[36]

By 1906, while Sioux Falls Lutheran Hospital had once again outgrown its building, local competition was encroaching. In addition to McKennan Hospital, in 1914 Dr. Moe of Minnesota built a small but

sophisticated hospital on 14th and Main streets that offered a variety of services including surgical, obstetrical and dental care. Because of the competition, instead of building a new structure, Sioux Falls Lutheran added a three-story addition at the cost of $30,000, which increased the hospital's capacity by another 30 beds.[37] Finally, in 1928, Sioux Falls Lutheran, recently renamed Sioux Valley Hospital, purchased land near 18th and Grange avenues; the hospital, today known as Sanford USD Medical Center, still occupies this site.[38]

Other medical facilities in Sioux Falls include the Royal C. Johnson's Veterans Memorial Hospital. The hospital was named for Royal C. Johnson who helped to create the Veterans Administration and was a South Dakota native. When it opened on July 24, 1949, Veterans Hospital was Sioux Falls' largest with 283 beds and, in addition to South Dakotans, it also served veterans from Minnesota and Iowa. In 1952, the "Crippled Children's Hospital and School" opened. While prior to this time the facility had been functioning for two decades as part of Sioux Valley Hospital, the polio epidemic of this era inspired supporters to campaign to have a separate, much needed facility built. The hospital expanded over the years and in 1994, it changed its name to Children's Care Hospital and School.[39]

McKennan Hospital

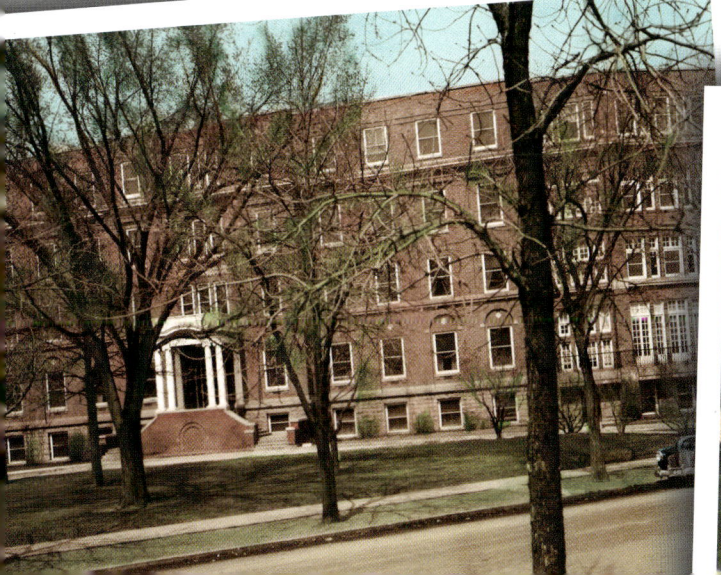

Veterans Hospital

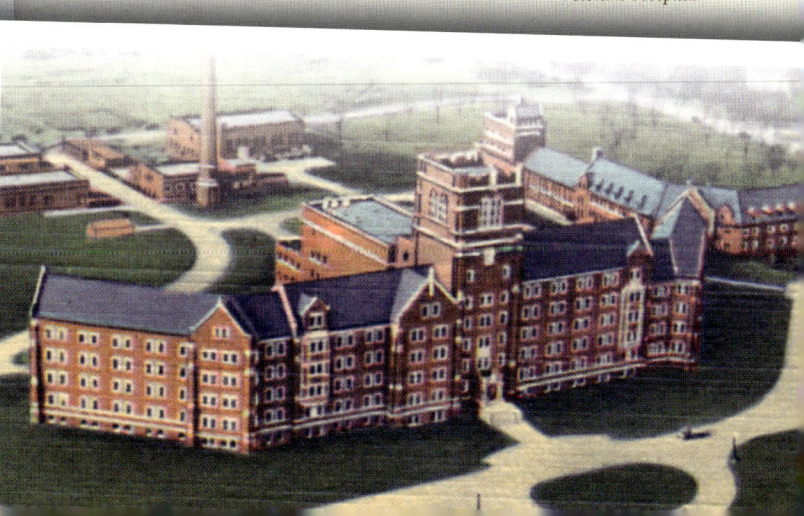

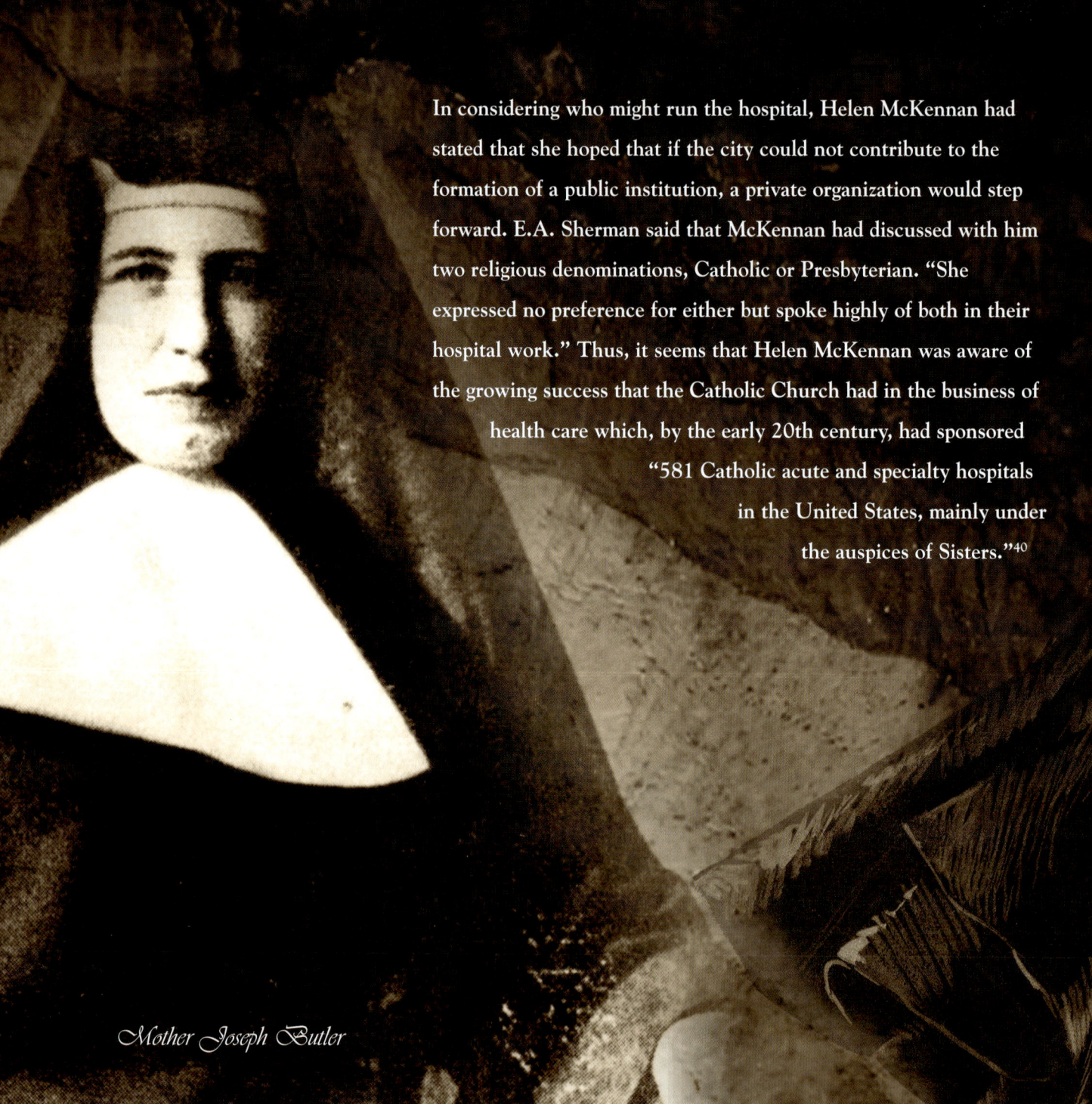

IRISH MISSIONARIES TO AMERICA

"... coming to help establish the much needed social services"

In considering who might run the hospital, Helen McKennan had stated that she hoped that if the city could not contribute to the formation of a public institution, a private organization would step forward. E.A. Sherman said that McKennan had discussed with him two religious denominations, Catholic or Presbyterian. "She expressed no preference for either but spoke highly of both in their hospital work." Thus, it seems that Helen McKennan was aware of the growing success that the Catholic Church had in the business of health care which, by the early 20th century, had sponsored "581 Catholic acute and specialty hospitals in the United States, mainly under the auspices of Sisters."[40]

Mother Joseph Butler

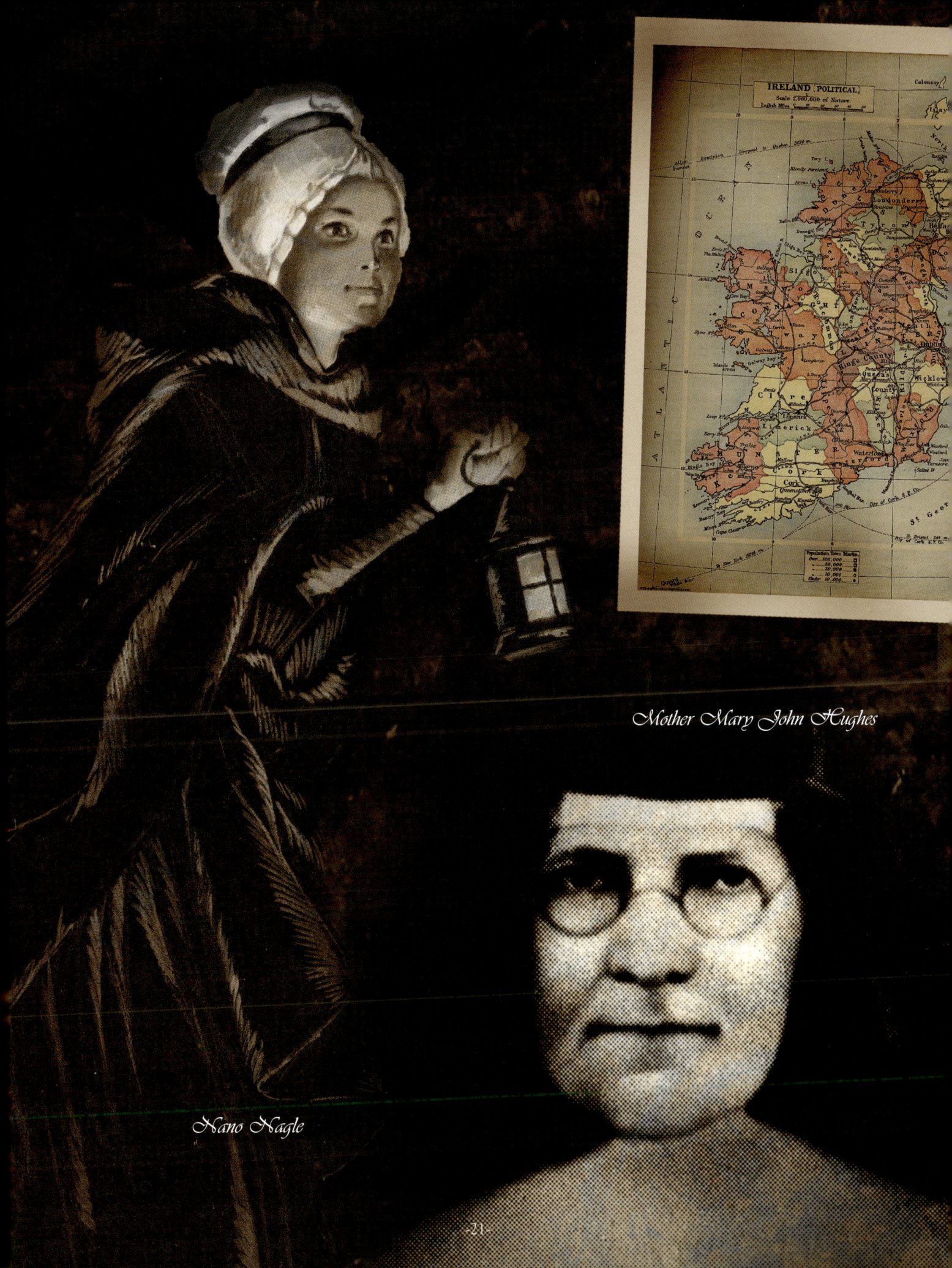

IRELAND (POLITICAL.)

Mother Mary John Hughes

Nano Nagle

"Our missioner seems in great spirits...

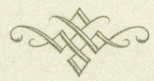

In 1906, at the time of Helen McKennan's death, in South Dakota the
Presentation Sisters were already operating two hospitals while the Benedictine
Sisters had opened Sacred Heart Hospital in Yankton in 1897. Like Helen
McKennan, few of the women of these communities were originally from South
Dakota. Most had been recruited from locales both national and international.

In the latter half of the 19th century, the United States opened its arms to
millions of immigrants and one small country sent many of its own as it wrestled
with economic hardship and natural disaster. As they fled the Great Famine of
the 1840s, the Irish had first settled in the urban northeast, but throughout the
19th century they steadily moved westward. As a result, by 1880, the Irish were
the third largest group in almost all western states.[41] Among these immigrants
were Catholic clergy and sisters who were coming to help establish the much
needed social services.

Among the women who left Ireland for the United States were the Presentation
Sisters, a religious order of women that Honoria Nagle, known as "Nano,"
founded in Cork, Ireland in 1791. Nagle, born in 1718, left Ireland at the age
of 13 to be educated in an Ursuline School in France. She returned to Cork
in 1749 and dedicated her life as a teacher to the poor children of the city.[42]
By the time of her death in 1784, Nagle had established a number of schools
and founded the Sisters of the Presentation of the Blessed Virgin Mary.
By the late 19th century, there were Presentation convents throughout Ireland
and beyond.[43]

Ireland's Presentation Sisters first arrived in the United States in 1854, with
five women establishing a convent in San Francisco, followed by another four
traveling to Dubuque, Iowa, in 1875. In January of 1880, Sister Bridget Carroll,
Mother Superior of the Presentation Convent in Dublin, Ireland, wrote to

... and hopes to be able to start for America with several companions early in March!"

Dublin's Roman Catholic Archbishop, Edward McCabe, that, "Our missioner seems in great spirits and hopes to be able to start for America with several companions early in March!"[44] The missioner, Mother Mary John Hughes, believed that she was called to work in North America where she hoped to found a Presentation convent. Mother John and her contingent arrived in the Dakotas in 1880, and eventually made their way to Fargo where she helped to establish St. Joseph's Convent.[45] Then, in 1886, Mother John led a small group south and opened the doors of a second Presentation convent and school in Aberdeen.[46]

After Mother John's return to Fargo in 1892, the Aberdeen Sisters continued with their education agenda; however, in 1900 circumstances caused their mission to broaden. There, as a diphtheria epidemic threatened, Mother Joseph Butler, Superior since 1894, immediately offered part of the convent as a place to nurse the sick.[47] Within a year, the Sisters had built St. Luke's Hospital and quickly found themselves laying the foundations for the largest Catholic health care system in South Dakota.[48]

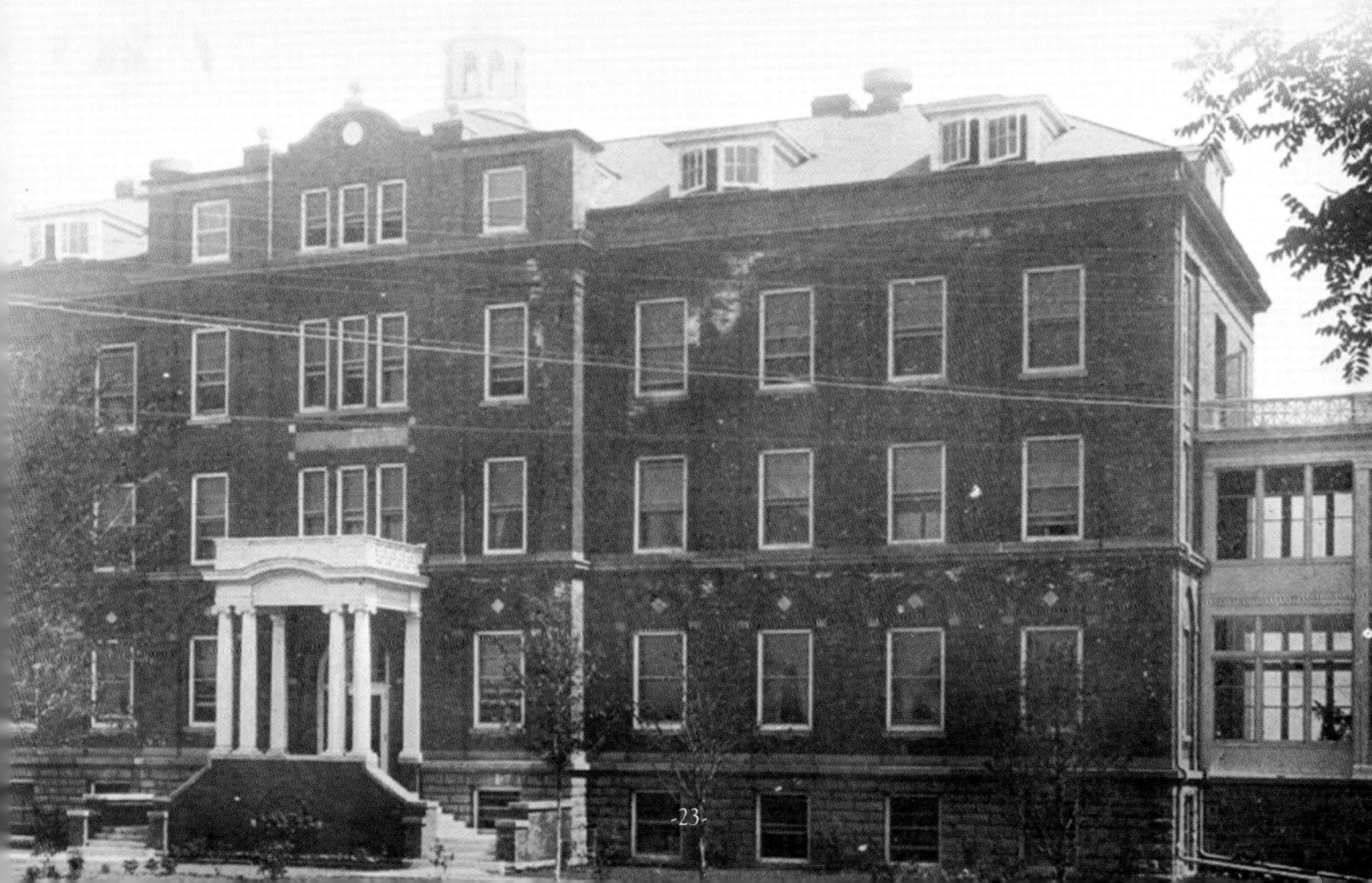

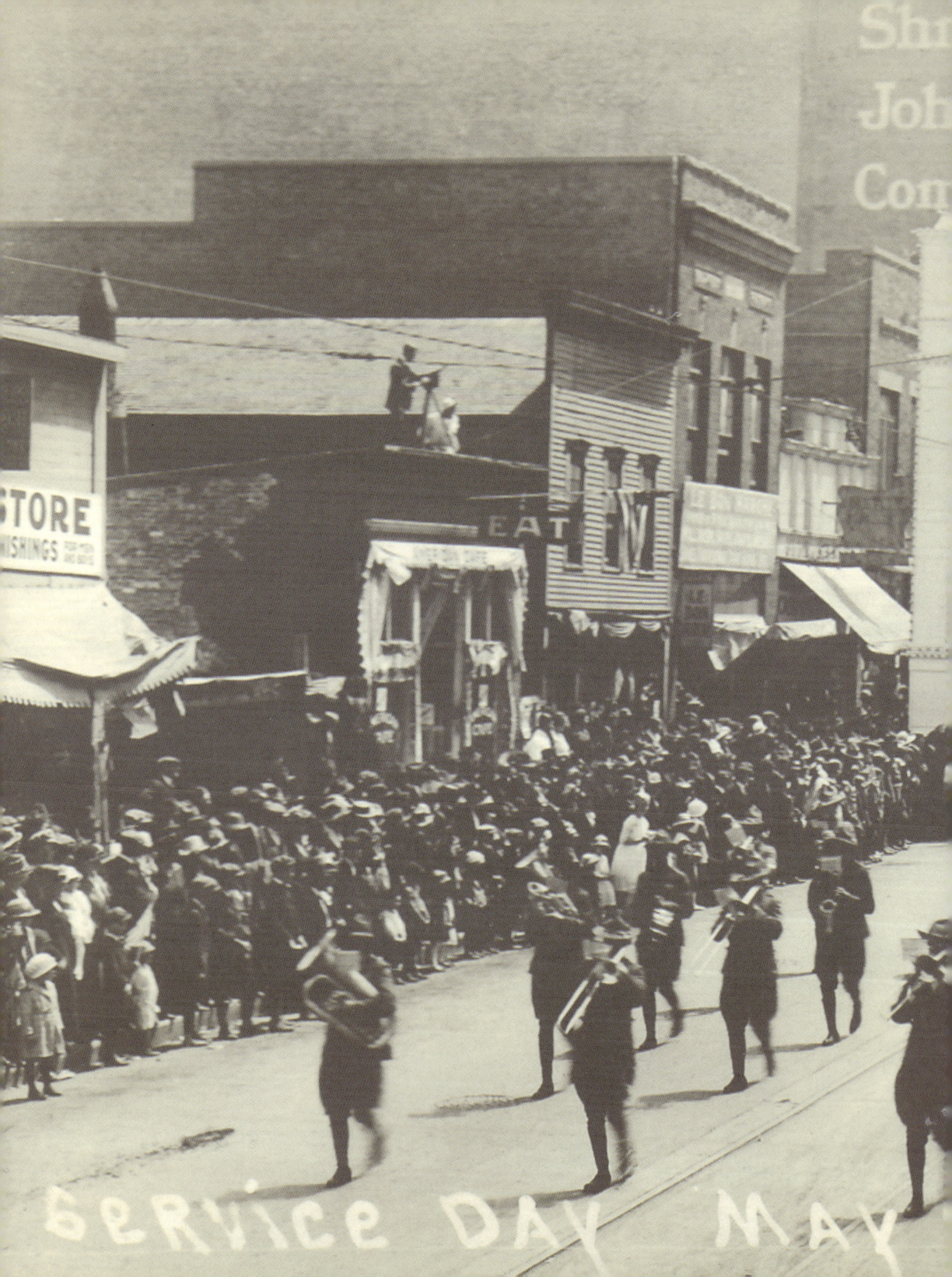

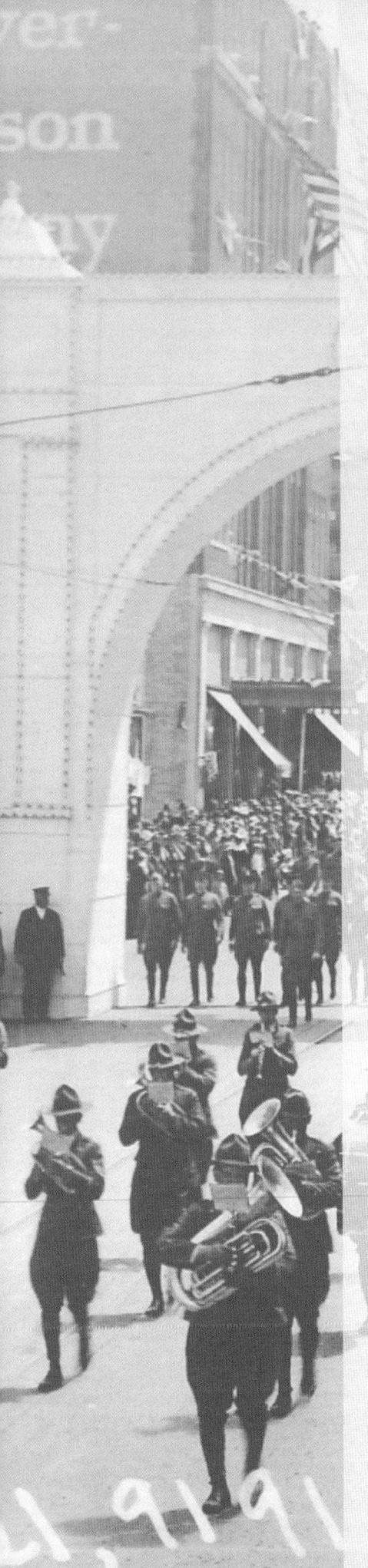

McKennan Hospital's Early Years and the Spanish Flu

Immediately after McKennan Hospital opened, the institution struggled because costs outpaced income and, as a result, the trustees had to borrow money to meet hospital expenses. During its first year, McKennan Hospital welcomed only 100 patients, but the numbers picked up and by 1916 McKennan had served over 1,000 patients. The annual report of 1916 particularly noted that not only was McKennan Hospital attracting the citizens of the city, but clearly persons from miles outside were arriving at its door for care.[49]

During this time, Sioux Falls, like the rest of the United States watched as the world entered into World War I. On June 29, 1914, the *Argus Leader* reported that Archduke Franz Ferdinand and his wife were assassinated in Serbia, foreshadowing the beginning of World War I in August of that year.[50] While the United States sought to remain neutral, it nevertheless provided support to Britain and France and, as a result, was increasingly drawn into the war. On April 6, 1917, the *Argus Leader* declared "U.S. Enters World War; German Ships Seized" reporting that the United States planned to draft 500,000 men during the coming summer.[51]

In addition to the enemy on the Western Front, there was another battle that was being waged—this one throughout the world and against an enemy that would be a much greater challenge than the German army. On March 7, 1918, the *Argus Leader* featured an article titled "Sammies Have No Epidemics." While the story stated that the American Army was proud of the fact that it was dealing with low rates of venereal disease among the soldiers, it noted that pneumonia had "done the most damage, more in fact than all other agencies, germ or German, combined."[52]

Nevertheless, this article was clearly indicating something more foreboding. Just as a month before, the *Argus Leader* reported that a deadly plague was sweeping China and that few of its victims had survived with over 40,000 dead in Mongolia alone. This "plague" was likely the flu pandemic which encircled the globe at the end of World War I. Even though what became known as the "Spanish Flu" continues to challenge scientists, recent research suggests that in addition to the influenza virus, a second "bacterial infection led to most of the deaths during the 1918-1919 pandemic."[53]

As the highly contagious flu outbreak began to spread, by the spring of 1918, the United States was quarantining its military bases. The flu's progress can be seen through the *Argus Leader*. In September 18, 1918, it featured a reassuring article that suggested that despite cases of influenza arriving on a ship docked in New York, the death rate at that time in New York was half what it was the prior year.[54] However, on September 25, the news quickly changed as the *Argus Leader* stated that the "Spanish Grip is Spreading Rapidly [in the] East" with calls by federal and state officials for more effective measures to fight the flu. The next day, September 26, the paper described how the influenza had spread to Army camps, and that the government was now mobilizing medical and nursing units for those areas of the country where the epidemic had "gained considerable headway." On October 3, the *Argus Leader* reported that flu cases for the Army were on the decline but it was "rapidly spreading among the civilian population…the malady has appeared now in 43 states and the District of Columbia."[55]

The news hit much closer to home when on October 8 the paper announced that Pierre and Sioux City had closed schools. The Red Cross was mobilizing forces to combat the contagion and enrolling nurses who would "freely use its accumulated hospital supplies to fight the epidemic." Next, on October 12, the *Argus Leader* stated that local authorities had issued "sweeping orders effective at noon today, closing practically everything in Minnehaha County. Churches, all public meetings, theaters, movies and every place where crowds assemble in or outdoors are barred until further orders."[56]

As scholars reflect upon the flu, they describe that it appears to have arrived in waves, the first in the spring of 1918 being less deadly than those that followed. Persons who were sick with the earlier bout, researchers suspect, may have been protected against the ravages of the later influenza. As a result, the strain of 1918 was particularly virulent to those aged 20 to 40, and less so for the very young and elderly. The death toll for the Spanish Flu is estimated to be as high as 25 million worldwide, and in the United States it appears that a quarter of the population became sick with some 675,000 dying as a result; this is more Americans than U.S. soldiers who died in combat in World War I, World War II, Korea and Vietnam combined.[57]

In South Dakota in 1918 influenza killed 1,847, "whereas in the year 1917 only 54 people succumbed to the malady," the *Argus Leader* reported. In truth the numbers for 1918 were probably higher as Pierre's Vital Statistics Bureau did not include the 544 who died of pneumonia.[58] Throughout the state, flu cases challenged the resources of all hospitals. McKennan, between September of 1918 and March of 1919, listed 173 with the virus, though that number was likely higher as those with pneumonia, not included in the count, had probably contracted the flu.[59] As one McKennan nurse recollected, patients came to the hospital "already black-looking from the high temperature, and many were in the last stage of pneumonia. I worked three weeks all day except for three hours off. Fifteen of the student nurses were ill, none died, but some lost their hair. I helped the undertaker carry out the bodies, there were so many."[60] The epidemic, which forced the hospital to place patient beds in hallways, made clear what McKennan's administrators already knew: the hospital needed to expand. Well before the pandemic, McKennan's leadership watched as rising patient numbers pushed the hospital's limits. The hospital cared for fewer than 500 in 1912, but by 1918 had annual admissions of over 1,300.[61]

The hospital had also made steady gains financially and proudly announced that it had cancelled $25,000 in outstanding bonds; Colonel Brown stated the money was not made through income but instead was "saved by the faithful women who are doing the work here."[62] In June of 1918, the *Argus Leader* featured an article detailing that bids had been taken for the construction of a new addition to McKennan Hospital. The *Argus* stated that McKennan hoped to have the building "enclosed this fall" so that the interior could be completed in the winter and ready for patients in the spring.

The paper reported that the new addition would be attached to the current building and the area that connected the two buildings would "serve as a solarium for convalescent patients." Noting that there had been much research done on the extension, the *Argus Leader* stated that once finished, "McKennan Hospital will be a thoroughly equipped hospital." In November, the paper revealed that the $160,000 addition was rapidly heading for completion and hoped to open on April 1, 1919. Once completed, "Sioux Falls will have one of the largest and best institutions of the kind in this part of the northwest." The five-story extension doubled the hospital's capacity and the addition added 76 beds which allowed the hospital to accommodate up to 131 patients. "It brought new room space for the medical, surgical and maternity departments and added obstetrical delivery rooms, a baby nursery and clinical laboratories," reported the *Argus Leader*.[63] This new building reflected the post-war nationwide changes which were directed toward providing the latest medical technology and particularly included a strong push to bring obstetrics into the hospital and out of the home.[64]

As a result of the expansion, in 1920 the American College of Surgeons awarded McKennan Hospital formal approval and it became one of South Dakota's first "Class A" institutions.[65] This was an impressive accomplishment given that when the ACS conducted a formal review in 1918, "less than one-seventh of the first group of hospitals of over 100 beds…could meet the standards."[66] By 1920, McKennan was caring for over 1,500 patients annually and during that year it had gross receipts of over $100,000. As McKennan Hospital anticipated its 10th anniversary, Helen McKennan's legacy was now sitting on a solid foundation.

A Legacy of Leadership
Mother Raphael McCarthy

Given that she placed her signature on all important transactions, in the first half of the 20th century, the convent's Mother Superior was effectively considered the president of a corporation that included the Presentation hospitals and schools. During McKennan Hospital's early history, it was the leadership of one Mother Superior in particular that was noteworthy.

Margaret McCarthy was born in Bandon, County Cork, Ireland on May 1, 1888. In 1907, Mother Joseph Butler recruited Margaret to the religious community during one of her recruiting trips to Ireland and Margaret, taking the name Raphael, entered the novitiate in South Dakota in 1908. Eventually, Sr. Raphael trained as a nurse and worked in Aberdeen's St. Luke's Hospital and, while there, after showing talent in administration was "assigned to the office of superintendent from 1913-1921."[67] As the Presentation hospitals struggled through the events of the early 20th century, the Presentation Order's records offer a glimpse at how Sr. Raphael's management savvy allowed her to strengthen the Presentation Order's ability to continue in the businesses of education and health care in South Dakota.

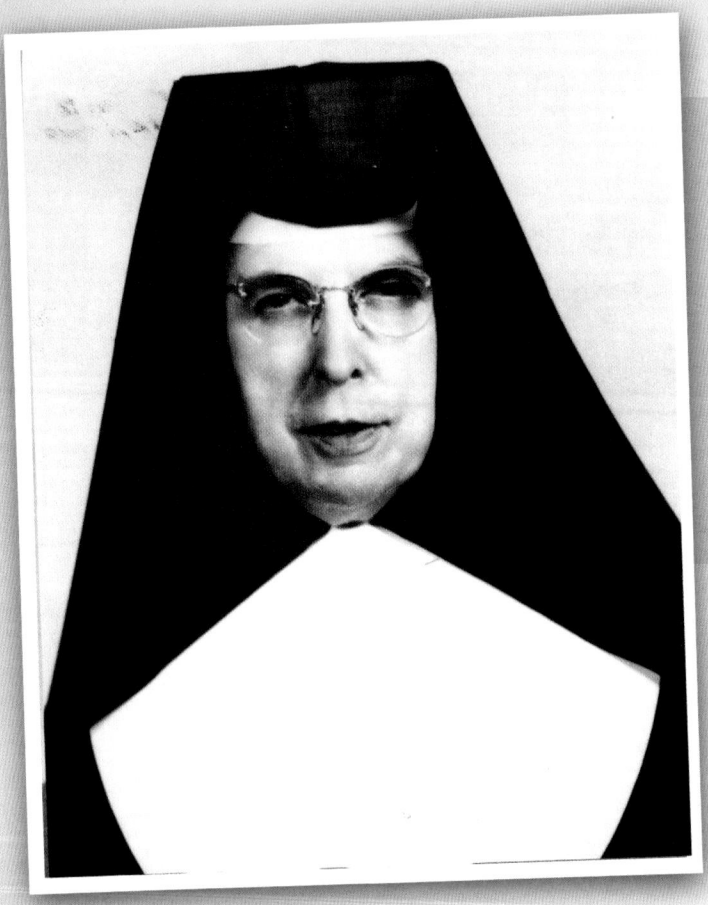

Sr. Raphael's business acumen soon became apparent when in 1925 she suggested the Presentation Order seek a loan for McKennan Hospital from Massachusetts Mutual Life Insurance, which she learned was offering money at a lower interest rate. There was, however, a catch. Mass Mutual stated that it would only offer the loan if the Presentation Order took full control of McKennan Hospital and accept the loan's risk. By 1925, the Presentation Order, like many Catholic Orders throughout the United States, had a solid financial track record. Thus, on May 5, 1925, Presentation Sisters Incorporated took full responsibility for McKennan Hospital and promptly negotiated a loan for $235,000.[68]

In 1927, Sister Raphael became superior-administrator of McKennan Hospital, the Presentation's largest hospital, which, like many local hospitals, was fiscally challenged. As one former nurse noted, Sister Raphael had confided in her that "she ran McKennan Hospital—food, lights, fuel, everything—on a budget of $8,000 per month."[69] Nevertheless, by 1932, the order had elected her Mother Superior and now she had a convent, all of its schools and four hospitals to run.

As Mother Superior she was, in effect, CEO of a company that had at that time 192 Sisters and employed many more lay persons in its schools and hospitals.

Not long after assuming her leadership role for the convent and hospitals, Mother Raphael established a uniform bookkeeping system that helped clarify and organize the order's financial position.[70]

In looking at some of Mother Raphael's extant letters we see a woman who understood the financial complexity of the businesses she ran while facing impressive odds. In 1934, in the midst of the Great Depression, Mother Raphael wrote to the vice president of Massachusetts Mutual stating that she was sending $10,000 toward McKennan Hospital's loan and this despite "the drought and the grasshoppers…and the inability of so many of our customers to pay their obligations to us…[these] have caused us to be in… financial difficulties."[71]

McKennan faced the same challenges that many hospitals in the United States were experiencing as, on average, U.S. hospital receipts per patient "fell from $236 to $59 between 1929 and 1930; occupancy fell from 71 to 64 percent; and average deficits rose from 15 percent to 20 percent of disbursements."[72] In spite of these problems, Mother Raphael proudly spoke of being able to continue to meet her financial obligations and thanked Mass Mutual for reducing the interest rate on the loan.[73] Two years later, and clearly on top of things, Mother Raphael wrote to the cashier of Mass Mutual on April 23 regarding the loan stating: "I notice you have charged me for accrued interest… this is entirely contrary to our agreement with your home office…according to their figures we were to pay $2,700 per month until July 1st 1936, at which time all the interest due… would be fully paid up."

She went on to state that "we have complied with the arrangement in every way and are amazed" that Massachusetts Mutual would imply that there was an unpaid balance of $236.32.[74] That same year Mother Raphael asked again to have the interest rate on her loan maintained at 4.5 percent and not returned to the company's suggested rate of 5.5 percent. "Our situation in South Dakota the present year is the worst in our history. There is absolutely no feed of any kind left... I can see little hope of any income during the coming year." Mother Raphael noted in the letter that she was very grateful for all of Mass Mutual's support and "as proof of our good faith we hope to be able to pay in the neighborhood of $15,000" toward the loan's principal.[75] As the 1930s came to an end and the world again faced war, Mother Raphael regularly sent Mass Mutual money.

In 1942, with the United States well involved in World War II, Mother Raphael again sought to negotiate a loan for her various businesses; this time with Northwestern Mutual Life Insurance Company. Neil Gleason, who represented the convent's interests, expressed his support for her application despite some missing documentation and said "that if it were not for my faith in the Presentation Sisters, their excellent institutions and your leadership, I would be rather reluctant to pass upon these statements as submitted."[76] Mother Raphael responded with an apology for the missing documentation stating that she thought only the information on the hospitals, not for the motherhouse and schools, was needed. Within the letter she argued her case noting that they were a good risk despite the bills receivable for the hospitals being larger than they might have been in other places.

She noted "we live in a farming country and these bills are paid depending upon crop condition" and while the hospitals make every effort to collect, "so much drought and poor crops" have challenged people's ability to pay. On December 15, 1942, Gleason wrote to confirm the positive outcome of the application and requested that she, "as president of the respective corporations," sign the papers for the three loans at 3.25 percent interest rate: these loans were $190,000 on Presentation Academy of Aberdeen, $98,000 on St. Joseph's Hospital in Mitchell and $180,000 on Presentation Sisters, Incorporated for McKennan Hospital in Sioux Falls; a total of $468,000, which, in today's dollars is the equivalent of borrowing nearly $18 million.[77]

As was her habit, Mother Raphael began immediate repayment on the loans and over the next two years, she was able to make "substantial" installments—particularly, it appears, on the largest—that being the loan on property in Aberdeen. So substantial were her payments that in 1944, Mr. Gleason wrote to inform Mother Raphael that Northwestern Mutual was challenged by her plan to significantly reduce the principal on the Aberdeen loan. Gleason suggested that, instead, Northwestern Mutual "might be more favorably impressed if some portion of the sum could be applied on the Mitchell and Sioux Falls loans" since reducing the Aberdeen loan would result in a considerable loss to the company. Gleason noted that Northwestern had provided this low interest rate to many Catholic hospitals and these same organizations were paying back greater sums than Northwestern had counted on; consequently, Northwestern Mutual could not continue to accept such large repayment without penalty. As Gleason noted, "the situation has become acute and they cannot ignore the interests of policyholders." Gleason revealed that while Northwestern took responsibility for not anticipating borrowers' substantially increased incomes, at the same time, "they cannot ignore their responsibilities." As a result, Northwestern began to administer a 2 percent service charge on excess payments.[78] This did not deter Mother Raphael and in a letter from June of 1945, Gleason confirmed that she would make payments of $13,000 on the Aberdeen loan, $18,000 on McKennan's and $1,000 on St. Joseph's—all with a "premium of 2 percent." Nevertheless, Gleason expressed happiness at the reduction in indebtedness because this would make it "possible to undertake some of the other projects which you have been planning."[79]

In 1945, as the war came to an end, Mother Raphael made her most significant decision for the economic health of the Presentation Order itself; she purchased 100 acres in Aberdeen to eventually be the site of a new convent. In 1946, her term as Mother Superior ended; by this time the Presentation community now numbered 221 Sisters, owned over $2.3 million in land and property, ran four hospitals, 16 schools, and one junior college and had Sisters teaching in diocesan schools throughout eastern South Dakota and western Minnesota.[80]

Mother Raphael McCarthy died on July 3, 1966, but six years prior to her death South Dakota Senator Karl Mundt recognized Mother Raphael by noting her golden jubilee on August 11, 1960, in the

Congressional record. Included was a review of her life which noted both her "keen business sense" as well as her "moral efforts" to care for others in greater need.[81]

Finally, to further add to Mother Raphael's story, until a corneal transplant in 1961, she was effectively legally blind.[82] In an oral interview, Sister SaBina Joyce recalled that local architect, Howard Spitznagel, when told that Mother Raphael's corneal transplant had been successful stated, "We could never put anything over on her when she couldn't see." This was put more graciously by Sioux Falls Bishop Brady when in 1951, upon the 50th anniversary of St. Luke's Hospital in Aberdeen, he noted: "God has not blessed her with much sight in her eyes, but has given her the vision of a prophetess in her soul."[83]

Like her predecessors, Mother Raphael also traveled abroad to recruit women to the Presentation community in Aberdeen and during one of her trips to Ireland, Mother Raphael was approached by a young woman named Brigid Coakley. Born on December 28, 1927, Brigid Nodlaig* Coakley grew up in Cork, Ireland, one of three children of a Ford Motor Company employee and a homemaker. Brigid spent all of her school years at Cork's South Presentation School—site of the original Presentation convent. After graduating from high school, she attended Hynes School of Business in Cork and then got a job as a bookkeeper for Musgrave Brothers, a diversified company whose businesses included a laundry and wholesale/retail grocery business. Increasingly, Brigid found that she was not inspired by this job.

A LEGACY OF LEADERSHIP

Sister Colman Coakley

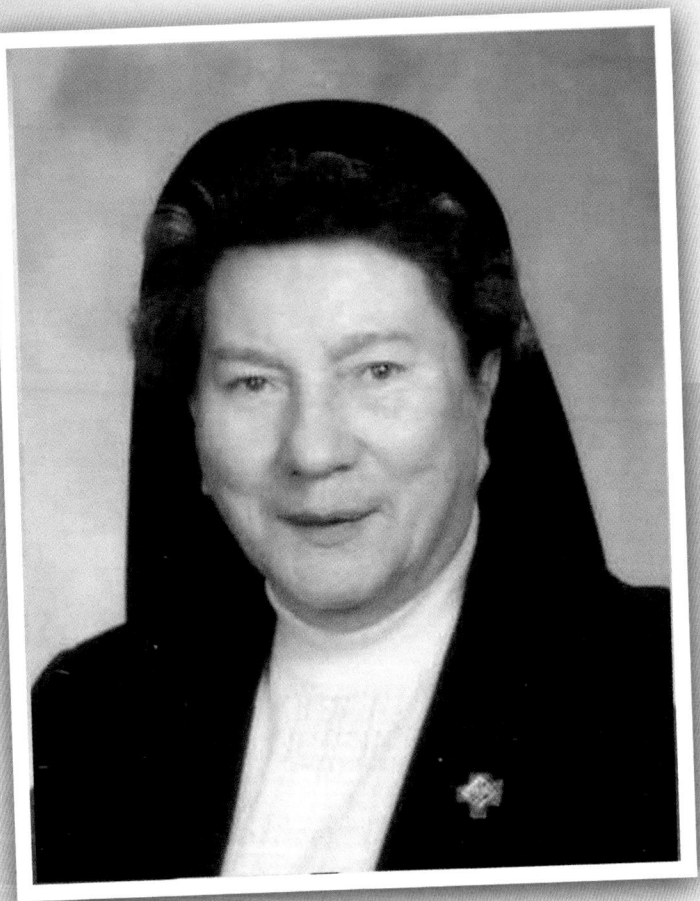

"I always thought I should be doing something better with my life," and thus, at about the age of 20, Coakley went to meet with Mother Raphael McCarthy during one of her recruiting trips to Ireland. The Presentation Sisters were imbued with the missionary spirit and Mother Raphael was no different; she inspired Brigid to accept her invitation to come to South Dakota and Brigid departed Cobh, Ireland, for a seven-day sea voyage to New York in May of 1949.

The novitiate took three years and in 1952 Brigid, now Sister Colman Coakley, arrived at McKennan to work for the Business Office. Sister Colman recalled with a laugh that:

The novitiate…was all study and preparation for the religious life. So I didn't know a nickel from a dime. Sister Borgia Fitzgerald, who was from Ireland, was in charge of the business office and she gave me a nickel, a dime and a quarter and told me to learn American money. And that was my introduction to the business office.

Thus, Sister Colman began her work in McKennan's business office and lived with the other Sisters in the basement of the 1911 hospital building. Part of her job included admitting patients. "Sometimes we had to take them to the emergency room. We acted as cashier, did insurance and payroll, took care of the switchboard and paid the bills. And all we had were adding machines and typewriters, and not even one apiece—we had to share."[84] Luella Ulin, who eventually became McKennan's accounting supervisor, remembered those Spartan conditions and noted that those who worked in the business office could just as likely be found taking care of patients or visitors because the business office was located at the hospital's front entrance. Ulin was told by Mother Cornelia Swanton, McKennan administrator during the 1950s, "The most important thing is the patient.

Make the patient feel comfortable and do your bookwork later."[85] It was Ulin who taught Sister Colman how to use the call system as well as the switchboard. Recalled Sister Colman:

> "The doctor's call system had been designed by Bishop Lambert Hoch and Louis Bouska. Bishop Hoch had been a chaplain at McKennan, and he was interested in engineering. The call system was a bunch of colored light bulbs in the hall up near the ceiling. Each doctor had a code, such as two flashes on red or three flashes on yellow. You just hoped that whoever it was would answer the light. I also had to learn the switchboard. I had an Irish accent so people couldn't understand what I was saying. I thought that it was the end of me. I have nightmares over that switchboard."

Most of all, what Sister Colman feared was taking OB patients up the elevator. "I was afraid they might deliver."

Sister Colman survived the trials of her early days and went on to take a series of leadership positions at the hospital. From 1958-68, she was the business manager.

"I remember when we got the first bookkeeping machine to do the payroll and to pay the bills. I thought I was in heaven. Otherwise, we were writing all the payroll checks by hand."

In 1968 she was named health care coordinator of all the Presentation Sisters' health care ministries and became chair of the Presentation Sisters' first Health Care Council—an organization which coordinated all of the Presentation health care ministries.

In 1972 she became the Director of Pastoral Care, a new department in the hospital. Sister Colman feels that this addition "fulfilled part of the total philosophy—the department ministers to the spiritual needs of the patients and family." Between 1970 and 1989, she was chair of the McKennan Hospital's Board of Trustees while in 1978, Sister Colman was named the first President of Presentation Health Systems. She became Chairperson of PHS in 1989, a position she held until she retired in 1996.[86] Along the way, Sister Colman, who had an associate's degree from Presentation College, completed her bachelor's in business at Augustana College in Sioux Falls.

McKennan Hospital grew from 278 beds to over 400 under Sister Colman's leadership.

John Hughes, former chairman of the hospital's Board of Trustees and a self-professed "big fan of Sister Colman's," stated unequivocally that Sister Colman was a very capable leader of the hospital and a "major player" in its growth and development. Paul Connelly, former board member and chair, reflected that she "was in tune with the mission of the hospital."[87] The late Don Bierle, a South Dakota senator and legal advisor to McKennan Hospital, reflected that Sister Colman shaped the Presentation Health System and improved quality while lowering costs.[88] Bierle added "Sister Colman is the one who makes sure the hospital and the health care system remember their mission."

Sister Colman echoed Connelly and Bierle in an interview she conducted in the early 1980s that "the mission of the Presentation Health System (PHS) is to provide a healing ministry to the sick, the elderly and the oppressed." At the system level Sister Colman's attention went beyond the Presentation-owned hospitals and focused on the health care needs of the entire region. By sharing the resources of PHS with small community hospitals she worked to improve health care in the more rural areas of South Dakota. This was emphasized when, in 1997, she was inducted into the South Dakota Hall of Fame as her nomination stated "her influence in the region will be felt for decades to come because of her efforts to strengthen health care in rural communities and because of the programs she developed to assure that Christian, gospel-based values in caring for the sick would be perpetuated."[89]

Sister Colman retired in 1996 and to the present she continues to watch over McKennan Hospital from her home that sits just across the street.[90] In July of 2010, Sister Colman Coakley celebrated 60 years as a member of the Sisters of the Presentation of the Blessed Virgin Mary. Of her life in health care ministry Sr. Colman noted that it "provided me with many challenges and opportunities to serve God by ministering to the needs of the people."[91]

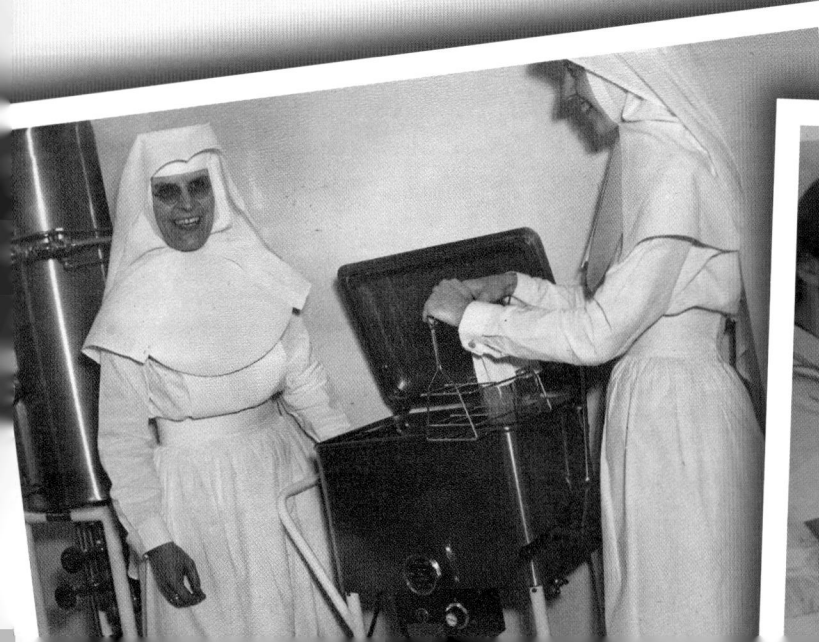

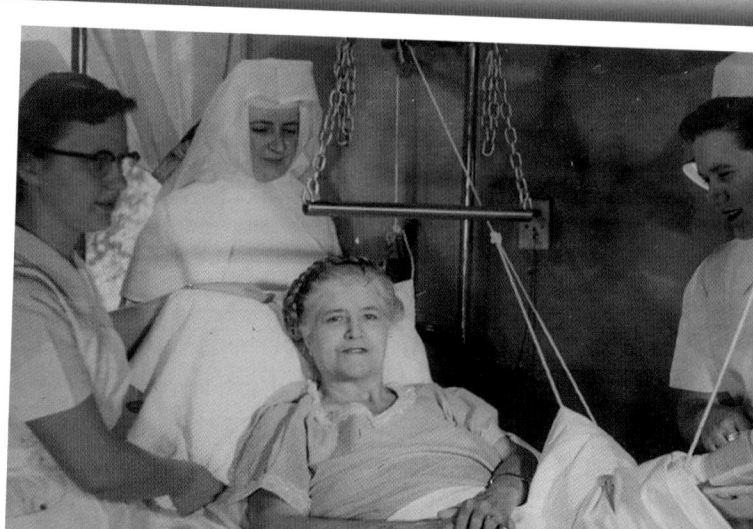

Nursing As A Profession

As the scientific understanding of medicine improved during the 19th century, the nursing profession also underwent a transformation. These changes came as the result of a variety of factors including an increase in the number of hospitals and medical facilities established to cater to the poor, a call for nurses during the Crimean and U.S. Civil Wars*, the increase in middle-class women's involvement in philanthropy and the sanitary reform movement which was part of the philanthropic agenda.[92]

As Bishop O'Gorman noted in his dedication of McKennan Hospital, women had distinguished themselves as nurses in the Civil War and had proven the benefits of the sanitary mission. As hospitals gained greater acceptance after 1870, the demands for improved training for nurses also increased and the three nursing schools in the United States in 1873 grew to over 1,000 by 1910.[93] Nurse training was arduous; students were expected to attend courses while also nursing patients and this made for long days with little free time. What little free time they had was often controlled by hospitals that generally housed nursing students on the premises. Many hospitals imposed strict curfews on nursing students—failure to comply could result in reprimand. Nevertheless, after World War II, institutions steadily sought to hire nurses with accredited medical training while diminishing their reliance on student nurses.

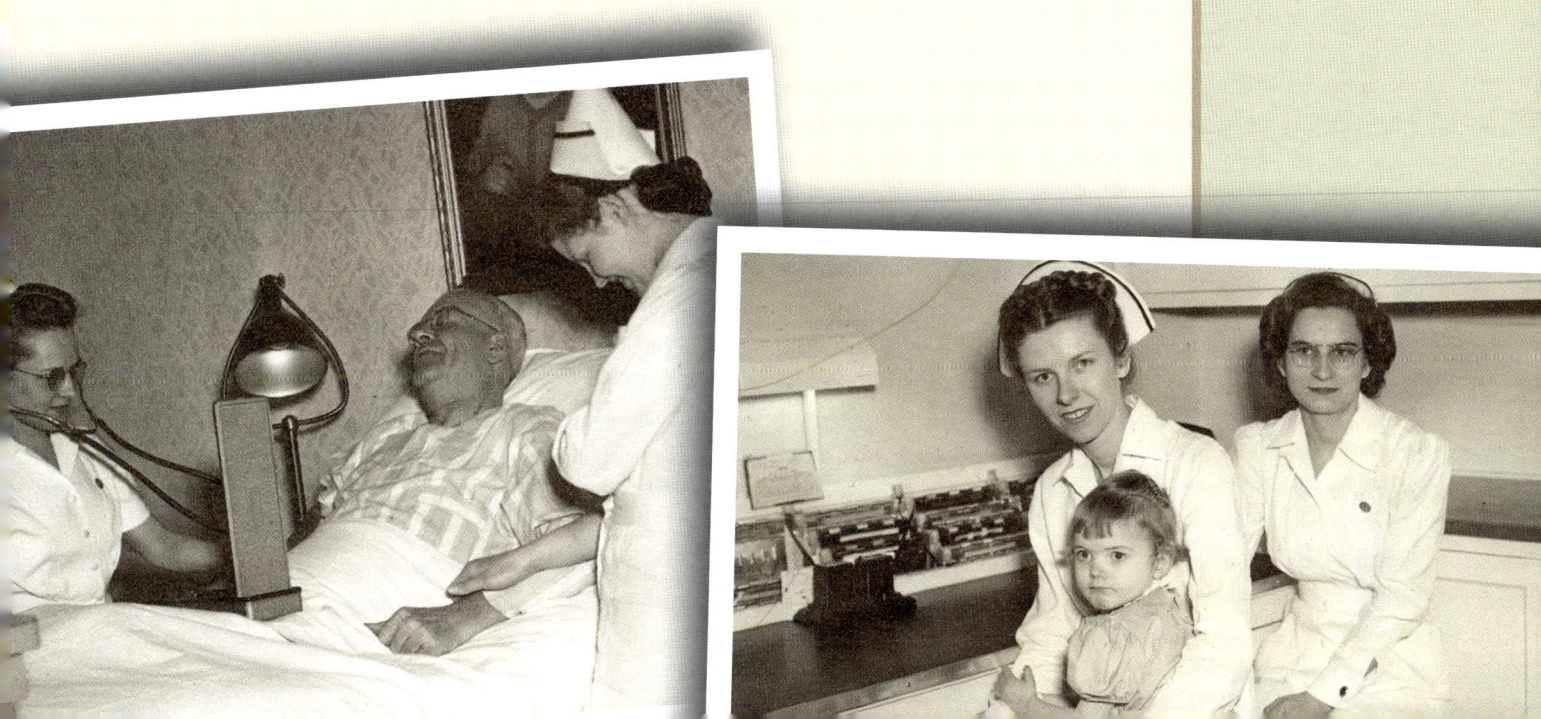

When McKennan Hospital opened in 1911, like the other three Presentation hospitals, it established a nursing school and welcomed its first students. Training was for three years, and while this would gradually improve, nurses' work was often as much housekeeper as medical attendant. As one of McKennan's early nursing students recollected, "The first month of training was mostly washing dishes. After that we were put on the floors [we were] assigned to bathe patients, change sheets, carry bedpans, and also do all the cleaning in the patient's room."[94]

The students spent much of the day in the hospital and went to classes late in the afternoon. A typical day was recalled by 1938 graduate Dorcas Baldwin:

> "We went to our stations in the hospital at 7 o'clock in the morning, and we were assigned patients. We had our lunch, came back and took care of our patients' noon meal and made sure that they were comfortable. We had class at 1:30 or 2:00 for about two hours. We were back down for our evening meal and ensuring that our patients had their evening tray, and then settled them for the night. And that was our routine, in other words, we worked for our tuition."

When Baldwin was a nursing student between 1935 and 1938, tuition was $50 for the three-year program; this paid for seven uniforms and books. The nursing students had a curfew of 11 p.m. on weekdays and midnight on weekends. Baldwin remembered that the nurses got an afternoon off every two or three weeks and were given an annual week's vacation. Many were from the country,

she recalled, and for some "it was the first time we had indoor plumbing." As Baldwin reflected, attending McKennan's nursing school was a great opportunity for many of the young women.[95]

A significant development for McKennan's nursing school came on July 1, 1943, when the United States, then involved in World War II, appropriated $45 million toward the Bolton Nurse Training Act which established the U.S. Cadet Nurse Corps. The act sought "to attract candidates to nursing and to give them recognition as national war workers."[96] In order to be accepted into the Nursing Corps, a student needed to have a high school diploma, be admitted to a nursing school that was part of the program and "agree to make her services available for military, or other Federal hospitals, or essential civilian nursing services for the duration of the present war." Among other things, the students were provided with monthly stipends, three uniforms and scholarships to cover all tuition and fees.[97]

Mother Raphael, the Presentation's Mother Superior, sent some of her Sisters to Washington to apply for the program. The obstacle: none of the Presentation nursing programs, now numbering four, met the attendance requirement the government expected. They needed to combine the schools so that each hospital's nurse training program would be considered a branch of a central school in Aberdeen.

Not long after the Presentation Central School of Nursing was established, it began a publication titled the *Presentation Nurse* that followed the progress of the Nursing Corps program and offered insight into

Doing so within days of the deadline, in 1942, the newly established Presentation Central School of Nursing was the

fourth school in the nation approved by the U. S. Cadet Nursing Corps.[98]

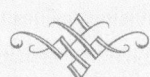

As part of this program, Presentation Central School of Nursing committed to accelerate the coursework for nurses and "reserve the last six months of training for service in the military or civilian hospitals that had greatest need."[99]

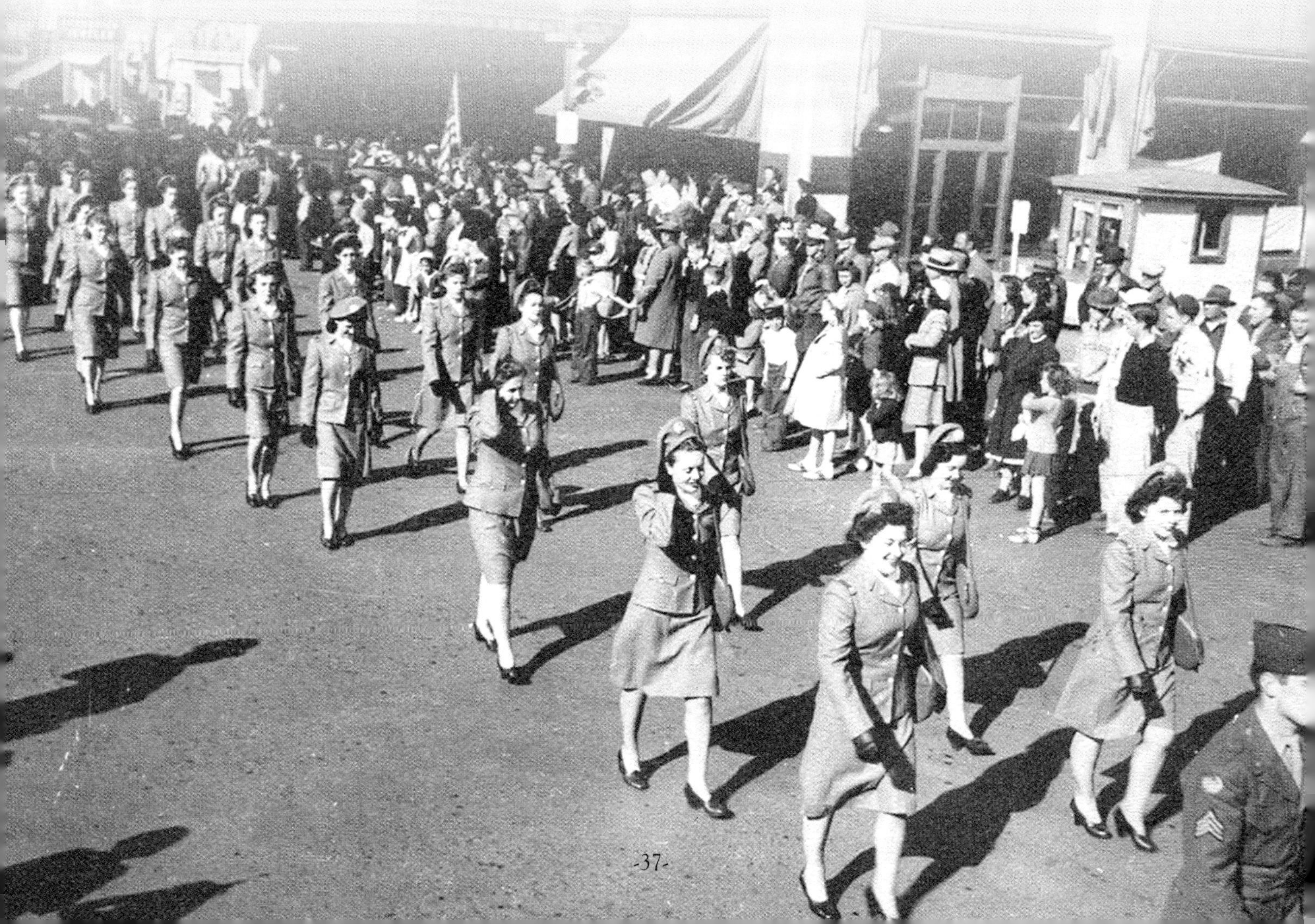

the increasing involvement by local nurses in the war. In February 1943, the *Presentation Nurse* told of how senior students were eligible to join the Red Cross, which then gave "the Army and Navy officials a better idea of the number of nurses available for the future." It announced that, as members of the Cadet Nursing Corps, these women were vital to the war effort but would also be vital after the war "in veterans' hospitals and in the rebuilding of civilian health service restricted by the war."[100] Congress appropriated over $176 million to the program in an effort to recruit and train more nurses and by the war's end, there were 57,000 nurses serving in the Army Nurse Corps.[101]

Another war-era change for McKennan's School of Nursing came in 1939 when the Sioux Falls Roman Catholic Diocese gave the hospital the Bishop's residence. Costing approximately $20,000 to build in 1890, the structure was the home of South Dakota's Roman Catholic Bishop and sat across from McKennan Hospital. Bishop William Brady donated the home to the hospital as reimbursement for care of ill priests that McKennan had provided over the years.[102] The home housed nursing students until 1968 when the McKennan School of Nursing closed.[103]

Like most hospitals of the time, McKennan Hospital almost solely relied on sisters and nursing students to provide nursing care. Nevertheless, as requirements for nursing care steadily grew more exacting, the hospital sought to adjust to the rising expectations placed on nurses. Sister Colman Coakley recalled watching the changes that came to nursing as there was an increasing call for students to spend more time in the classroom. "There was always this question whether the students were here for service or for education and it was always a kind of conflict."[104] Sister Colman was seeing the nationwide struggle over nursing education. Hospitals enjoyed the cheap labor of student nurses and were loath to let them reduce their nursing activities in order for them to spend more time in the classroom. However, as medicine became more sophisticated and as stricter educational standards were implemented, hospitals steadily decreased their reliance on students and began to hire fully trained nurses to care for patients.[105]

The McKennan Hospital School of Nursing and Presentation Junior College, which had opened in 1951, sought to adapt to the changes.[106] In 1957, Presentation Junior College's nursing program provided pre-clinical classes in Aberdeen while future nurses once again pursued their clinical experience at regional hospitals to which Presentation Junior College affiliated. Thus a student could complete clinical work at McKennan Hospital in medical, surgical, maternity and pediatric care while going to either Omaha or Yankton for psychiatric training and to Chamberlain for rural nursing.[107]

Pressures to improve nursing education escalated. In 1965, Presentation announced that it would discontinue its program at McKennan in Sioux Falls and, beginning in 1968, the nursing program was centered in Aberdeen. Thus, the McKennan Hospital School of Nursing, which had been in existence since 1911 and graduated over 1,000 nurses, shuttered its doors in 1968.[108] To the present, Avera* McKennan remains a site for future nurses from local schools to gain clinical and professional experience.

Into the 1970s and 1980s, the nursing profession continued to experience growing pains and wrestled with educational expectations, qualifications and image. In addition to stricter educational requirements, another continuing challenge for nursing was that salaries neither kept up with the increased training nor the greater demands that came with the job. At the 50th anniversary of McKennan School of Nursing's class of 1945, LaVonne Wright recollected that when she graduated she made $1 per hour while Dewis Ahlberg stated that her beginning salary was 85 cents an hour.[109] Over 40 years later an article in the *Argus Leader* suggested things were little improved; the paper discussed that first-time hospital nurses in South Dakota started at little more than $20,000 annually, a salary that the president of the South Dakota Nurses Association noted was much lower than for other professional positions. In addition, nurses working in nursing homes, clinics or offices were usually paid considerably less than their hospital counterparts.[110]

During the 1990s compensation for nurses steadily improved and as McKennan Hospital entered the 21st century, it recognized that nurses made up the largest percentage of employees within the hospital and, as a result, sought to show appreciation for their service. In 2001, Avera McKennan became the first hospital in South Dakota and only the 36th hospital in the nation to gain a "gold medal" for nursing excellence as a Magnet® hospital. The recognition was repeated in 2005 and again in 2009.[111] Fewer than 1 percent of hospitals in the country have achieved three consecutive recognitions through the Magnet Recognition Program® by the American Nurses Credentialing Center honoring hospitals that seek to provide a positive working environment and foster

quality nursing care. "If hospitals value nurses' input in decision-making, give them autonomy, and help them continue their development—if we encourage the best of the best—outcomes in patient care and quality follow," stated Carla Borchardt, director of professional nursing practice at Avera McKennan.

All of this comes with the recognition that nursing requires much of those who practice it. "Nursing is both an art and a science," said Avera McKennan's Judy Blauwet, senior vice president of Hospital Operations and chief nursing officer at Avera McKennan. "Our service in caring for patients is the art; our competence in providing quality care is the science."[112] Nevertheless, Blauwet suggested that it is easy to get caught up in the technology of medicine "but we can't do so at the expense of the personal connection…the relationship connection."[113]

Today, Blauwet thinks that a nursing career may be a key to opening many doors. A nurse for over 30 years, Blauwet has spent most of her career at Avera McKennan and has held a variety of positions in the hospital. Beginning in the ICU, where a part-time position allowed her to take care of her three children, she moved on to help in the implementation of the Meditech Nursing Module, became a director in the ICU area, and developed business plans for the hospital including the establishment of the Careflight* service. Eventually she became vice president for Business Development before moving into her current position. As Blauwet stated, a nursing degree can open the door to many career options: "Nursing is also a good background for health care law, finance, administration and clinical management."[114]

A Few of McKennan's Early Physicians

The first patient arrived at McKennan's doors on the day of the hospital's dedication and Dr. Gilbert G. Cottam was there to perform an emergency appendectomy. Born in England in 1873, Cottam moved to Sioux Falls in 1909 where he became chief of staff at McKennan Hospital.[115] He left Sioux Falls in 1939 to practice in Minneapolis, but returned to South Dakota in 1943 to be superintendent of the South Dakota Board of Health.[116] Cottam was one of a long line of compassionate physicians who cared for patients at McKennan Hospital.

Gilbert Cottam passed on his love of medicine to his son, Dr. Geoffrey I. Cottam. Geoffrey Cottam was born on April 21, 1897 and graduated from Washington High School in Sioux Falls; after which he served in the U.S. Calvary, Troop B, during the last year of World War I. He attended the University of South Dakota for his first two years of medical school and received his medical degree from the University of Iowa in 1926. After taking additional courses at Harvard University and working at Miller Hospital Clinic in St. Paul, Minn., he returned to Sioux Falls in 1931 and the next year entered into a partnership with Dr. S.A. Donahoe. Cottam spent his career performing groundbreaking surgery because, as he said, he hoped such advanced surgery would encourage more surgeons to come and practice in South Dakota. In 1933, Cottam operated on a patient at McKennan suffering from a brain tumor and it is believed that this was the first surgery of its kind in South Dakota.[117]

Cottam continued to perform groundbreaking surgery, but as the numbers of surgeries that physicians conducted increased, they soon recognized that during even relatively routine procedures, a patient's heart could suddenly stop. Though doctors found that heart massage could make a difference, there was hope that more could be done. At about the same time that heart massage was introduced, it was also recognized that a small electrical shock could restore the heart's rhythm and Cottam wanted such a device.[118]

In 1953, Cottam put in a call to Dr. V. Ronald Nelson, chairman of the Physics and Math Department at Augustana College. Nelson was an expert in electronics and Cottam was looking for someone to build him a "heart shocker." According to Nelson, Cottam called one Friday afternoon saying that on Monday he had a surgery scheduled for which he wanted a defibrillator. Nelson had no model to design from, but instead used information he gained from medical journals. With the help of assistant Gary Gledd, they began work on a defibrillator. Improvisation was needed. "For example, to make the spoon-like electrodes which the doctor places on the heart to close the circuit for the shock, they purchased regular kitchen spatulas. Putting their workshop to use they ground the metal to the desired shape and size and insulated the handles." This quick thinking cost Nelson $2.50. The next problem was ensuring that the medical staff was not also shocked as the patient lay on the stainless steel operating table. With this solved, by the end of the weekend the two men provided Cottam with a crude "heart shocker"—the first in South Dakota. Thankfully, the first defibrillator Nelson built was not needed. The following week, Nelson went to work on a second, more sophisticated model, to be provided to McKennan Hospital. Dr. Cottam paid for both of these machines, spending approximately $200 on each. As Cottam stated: "I do a large number of chest and lung operations where there is danger of heart stoppage or fibrillation and having one of these beside me will be an immense comfort."[119]

Eventually Nelson's heart shocker was put to use at McKennan Hospital. In January of 1958, a man from Hartford, S.D., experienced fibrillation during abdominal surgery. According to the *Argus Leader*, when the new device was used the patient "suffered no ill effects" and, as the newspaper reported, "saving of [his] life was due, to an important extent, to the inventive genius of Dr. V. Ronald Nelson... and his assistant Gary Gledd. The defibrillator served to slow the heart to a point where the surgeon could begin massage and bring about normal function of the organ." By this stage, Nelson's machine was kept in McKennan's operating room at all times.[120]

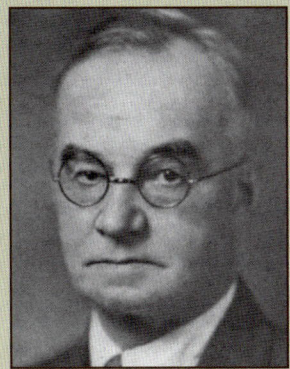

Dr. Geoffrey Cottam

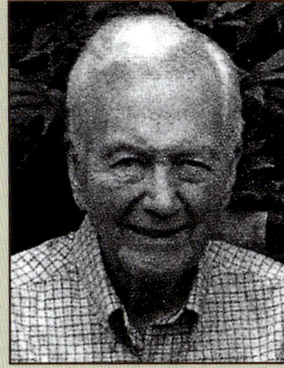

Dr. V. Ronald Nelson

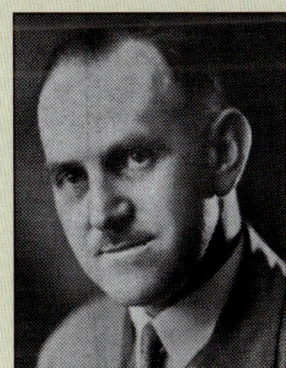

Dr. Will E. Donahoe

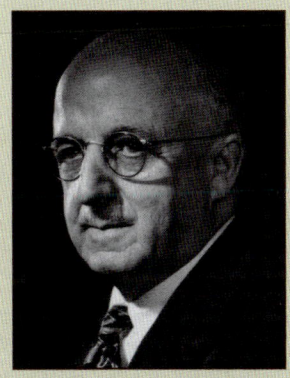

Dr. Guy E. Van Demark

Nelson continued to perfect his machine and, over the years, he supplied McKennan Hospital with refined versions. Many hospitals throughout South Dakota used Nelson's machine, helping to save countless lives.[121]

Another early practitioner at McKennan and a contemporary of Dr. Geoffrey Cottam's father was Dr. Will E. Donahoe. Donohoe, born May 18, 1886 and a long-time Sioux Falls resident, he became a pediatrician and sought to "keep children healthy but also to make them good citizens." A veteran of World War I, Donahoe graduated from St. Thomas College in St. Paul and received his medical degree from the University of Illinois in 1912. The following year, he helped to establish a clinic in Sioux Falls with his cousin Dr. S.A. Donahoe.[122] In 1919, Will Donahoe attended the University of Iowa for post-graduate studies in pediatrics and spent the rest of his career caring for children and advocating for improved public health. In 1920, Donahoe started the first free clinic for children in South Dakota.

Over the years, Dr. Donahoe contributed time to the Lutheran House of Mercy, the South Dakota Children's Home and the Presentation Children's Home.[123] In addition, Donahoe acted as chief of staff at both McKennan and Sioux Valley hospitals and between 1920 and 1931, Donahoe served as the Sioux Falls public school physician—free of charge. From 1936 to 1940, he was Sioux Falls' health officer as well as the superintendent of the County Board of Health. As health officer, Donahoe inspected at least 100 schools where he found deplorable conditions. As a result of his efforts, many schools renovated buildings to improve the environment.

At the 50th anniversary of McKennan Hospital, Dr. Donahoe wrote to Mother Viator Burns, Superior of McKennan Hospital, and reflected upon his affiliation with McKennan and his work with the Sisters.[124] "I have valued, as one of the blessings of my life, the privilege of association with you Sisters in my 49 years of medical practice," he wrote. Dr. Donahoe died at the age of 89 in December of 1975.[125]

Another early Sioux Falls doctor whose reputation is well known is Dr. Guy E. Van Demark. Born October 4, 1879, "in a claim shanty three miles north of Hartford, S.D.," Van Demark attended Northwestern University Medical School followed by an internship in Chicago. An orthopedic surgeon during World War I, Van Demark "pioneered and introduced many surgical operations in this area. He was the first doctor in Sioux Falls to treat fractured hips with hip pinning." In an *Argus Leader* profile, Van Demark noted that it was his time in the war that caused him to concentrate on orthopedics. A founding member of the Sioux Falls Medical and Surgical Clinic which opened in 1919 and located on Minnesota and 11th streets, Van Demark was a fellow of the American College of Surgeons and the American Academy of Orthopedic Surgeons.[126] Best known for his efforts to prevent deformities in children, he gained a regional reputation for his skill with particularly challenging cases. Van Demark tried to retire in 1949, but retirement eluded him as, along with his nephews Robert and Walter Van Demark who had entered into the practice with him, Van Demark's expertise remained in great demand. A bachelor nearly all his life, Dr. Guy Van Demark married only months before he died at the age of 84 on November 9, 1963.[127]

As these and other physicians helped to build Sioux Falls'
reputation for quality medical care, they attracted others who
desired to work in such an environment. In the years after
World War II, Helen McKennan's hospital

continued to maintain its quality of care
by hiring superior personnel as well as
expanding and improving its facilities.

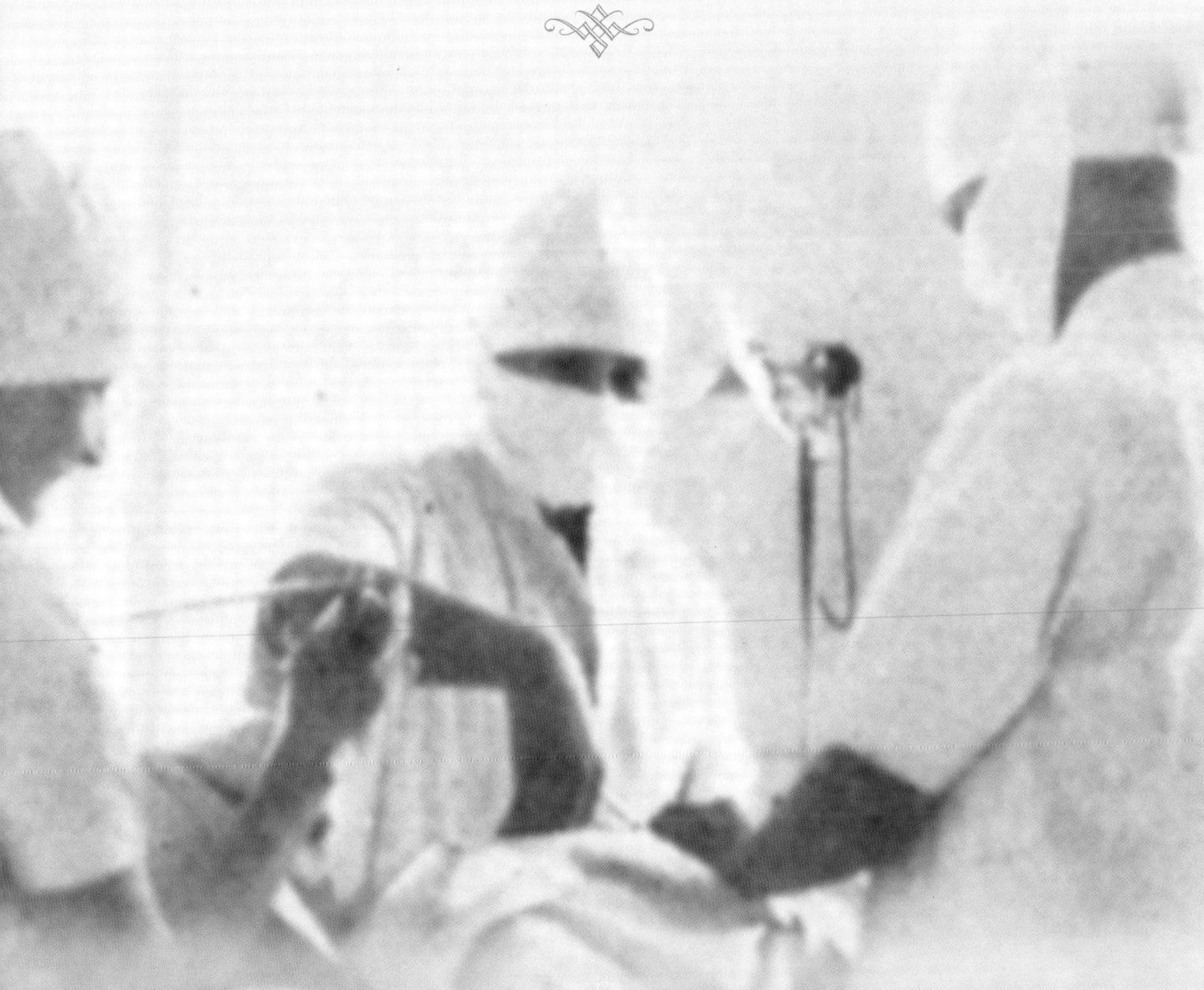

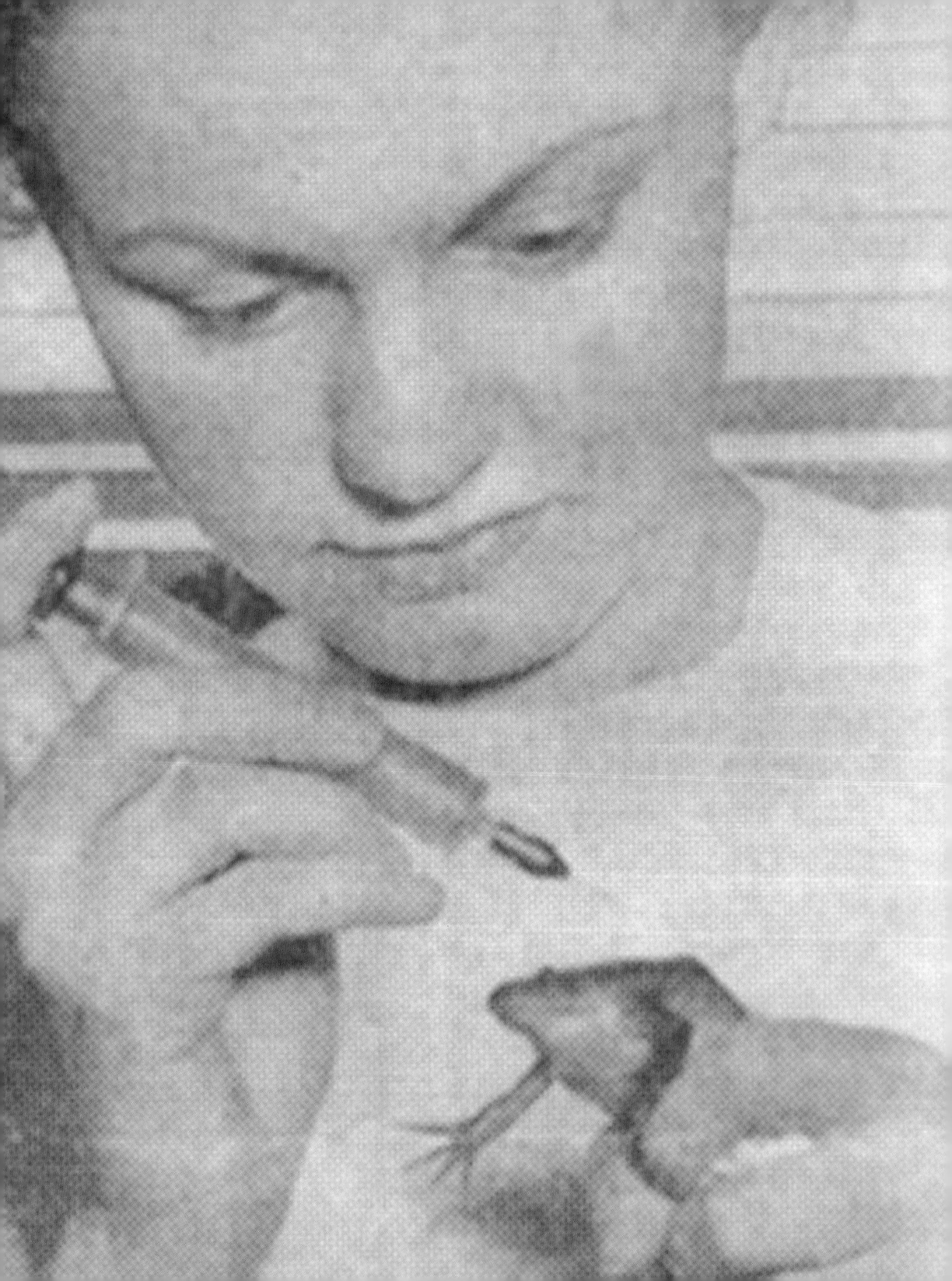

An Interesting Problem…

IN 1948, MCKENNAN'S LAB FOUND ITSELF WITH AN INTERESTING DILEMMA:
the hospital had run out of rabbits.

Every month McKennan went through approximately 25 rabbits in order to determine

pregnancy. Unfortunately for the bunny, it did not survive the test. When faced with

a lack of rabbits, McKennan Hospital authorities turned to a new species for help and

imported a number of South African clawed toad-frogs, the Xenopus Laevis, to do

the job. Good news for both rabbits and amphibians, the frogs survived the test.

In the late 1930s, Scottish Professor F.E. Crew had discovered that these creatures,

when injected with the woman's urine, would lay eggs if the woman was pregnant.

In addition, while the rabbit test usually took 48 or more hours, the frog provided its

news within a day. After a week's rest if negative, or a month off if positive, the frog

returned to the job of supplying happy news to many.

According to the *Argus Leader,* the biggest challenge for lab technicians was,

during the test, keeping a good grip on one of McKennan's new collection of $8 frogs.*

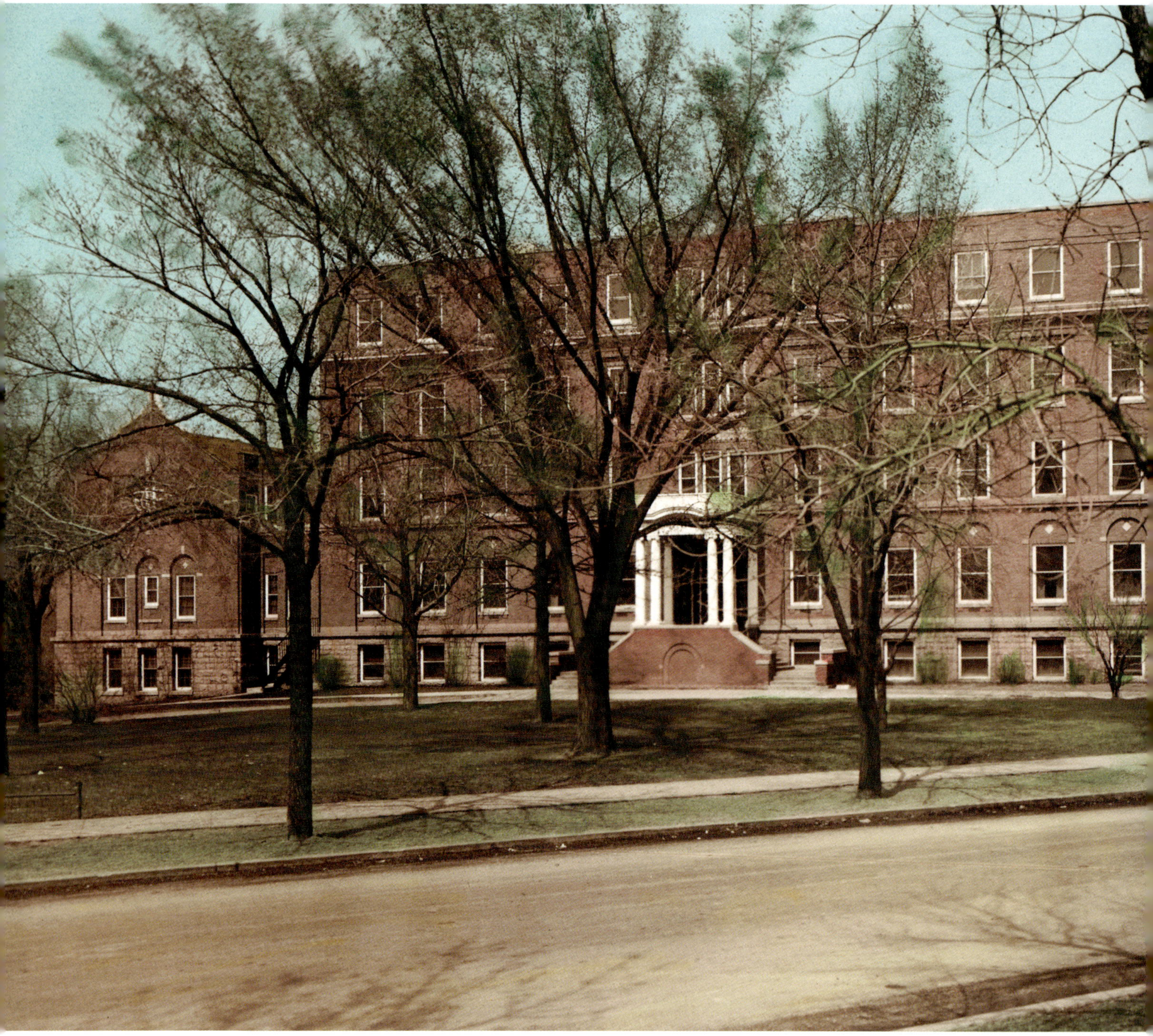

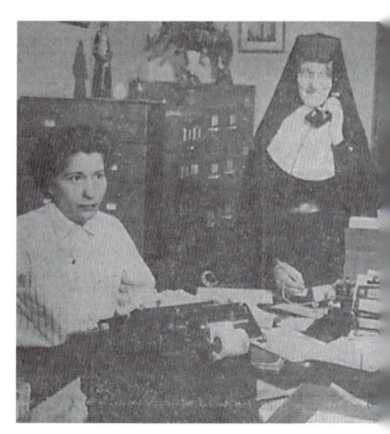

STEADY
GROWTH AND CHANGE

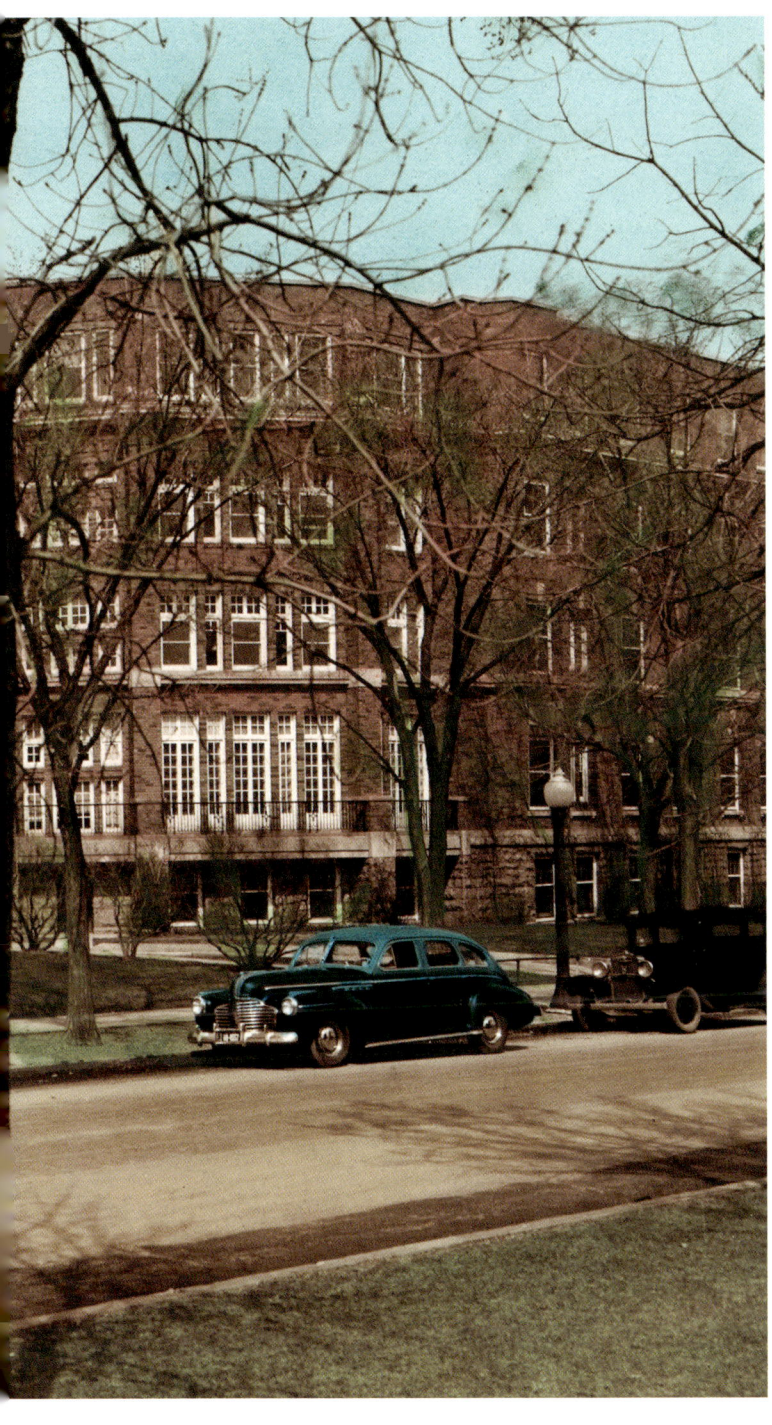

During World War II, Sioux Falls was host to an Army Air Corps Technical Training School. Established in 1942, the school trained thousands of servicemen and contributed to the city's growth. "As a result, the city experienced a frenzy of building unlike anything it had known since the frontier boom times of the 1880s."[128] The expansion included new manufacturing and other industries which then resulted in more homes, schools, churches and hospitals.

In the post-war years, the Presentation Sisters and McKennan Hospital sought to adjust to an increasingly sophisticated world. To begin, the Presentation Sisters recognized that they could achieve greater economies of scale through combining hospital purchases. Thus the Sisters reasoned that, for example, "if all four of their hospitals bought bed sheets from the same supplier…[it] might offer them a lower price." An agency called PACE (Presentation Affiliated Cooperative Effort) was born in 1946 and the Presentation Order centralized purchasing for all four hospitals. Under the guidance of Stan Costello who was based in Aberdeen, the Sisters "established one of the first successful group purchasing organizations in the United

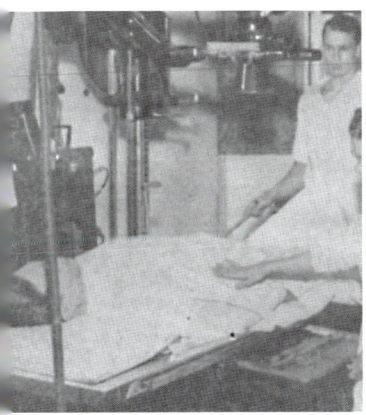
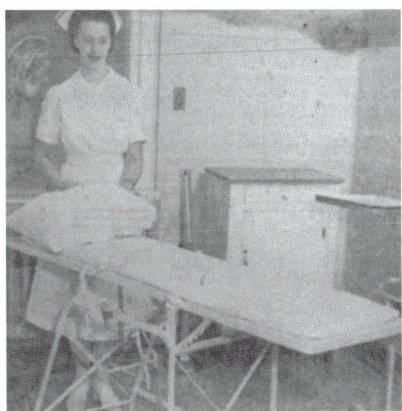
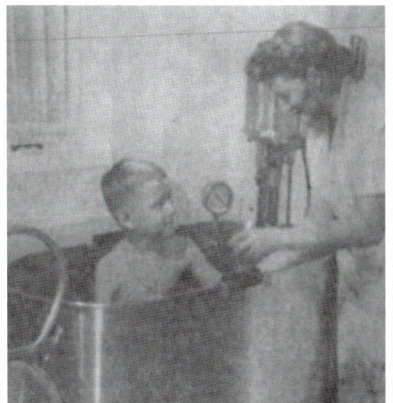
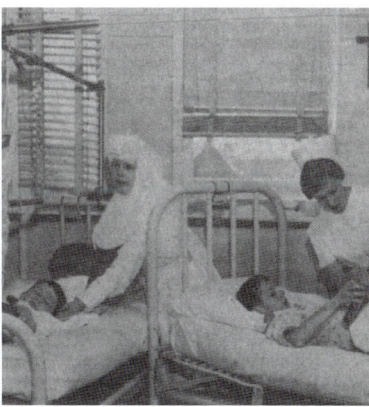

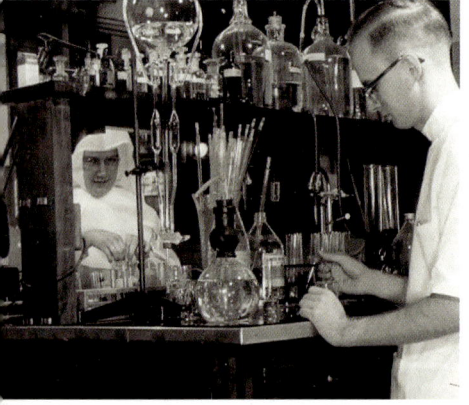

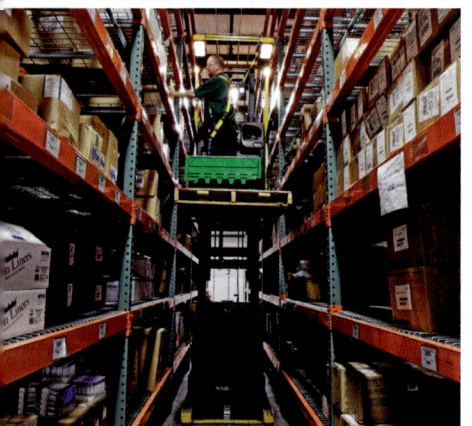

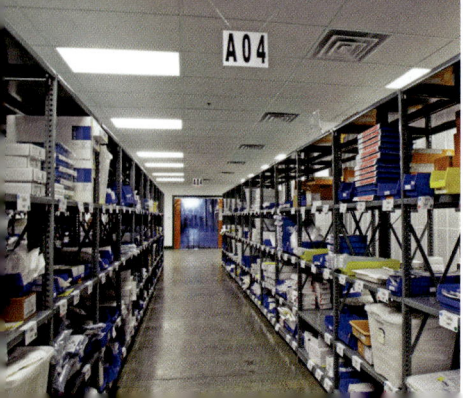

States." Costello continued to work with the Presentation Sisters and "from 1954 to 1976 increased PACE membership to 35 hospitals and about 200 other purchasers." In 1977, PACE officially incorporated and continued to broaden its services such that to the present it works with hospitals, clinics, surgical centers, long-term care facilities, and schools in South Dakota, Iowa, Nebraska, Minnesota and North Dakota.[129]

More significantly, by the mid-20th century, the world of medicine had become more scientific and technically sophisticated. Following World War I, better organized trauma care learned on the battlefield was applied in hospitals; during World War II, improvements, particularly in pharmaceuticals, brought other important advancements. Of these, the most noteworthy may have been Alexander Fleming's 1928 discovery of penicillin. The serum was not available for mass production until 1943, but widespread use of penicillin by military physicians enabled injured soldiers to be evacuated from the battlefield with decreased fear of infection. Such improvements quickly made their way into hospitals. In November of 1943, McKennan was the first hospital in South Dakota to use penicillin on a patient with a life-threatening staphylococcus infection. "Penicillin was first given [to the patient] on November 4, and the first blood culture taken one day later, showed that all staphylococci germs in the blood stream had been completely destroyed."[130] Hospitals had now become essential to medical care and, in the post-war years, they replaced the home as central to the provision of health care. The need for more hospital beds steadily increased and Congress sought to provide financial support to hospitals in order to fill in the gaps.[131]

At McKennan, support for expansion arrived in 1943 when it received a $49,637 federal grant to fund the hospital's need to remodel its fourth floor. The alterations included two new operating rooms, a laboratory and expanded pediatric department.[132] In these remodeled areas, McKennan made efforts to conserve space through improved technology including instrument sterilizers and steam-heated sheet and blanket warmers that were built into the walls. In addition to this large remodeling project, the hospital updated its facilities by offering such improvements as better access for ambulances, a library and improved carts for patient meals.[133] This reconstruction brought hospital capacity up to 180.[134] Nevertheless, McKennan Hospital continued to reflect the nation's need for more beds. It became clear that the 1911 and 1919 buildings were inadequate, both for patient needs as well as for accommodating the changing technology of medical care.

Space was tight. Nurse aid Kay Brink, and nurses LaVonne Gaspar and Margot Nelson each noted that there was a seven-bed room in which males with more minor medical problems were placed; the bathroom for the seven men was down the hall. In addition, Gaspar, who has been with McKennan for over 47 years and helped to establish the hospital's first coronary care unit, noted that the patients could smoke in their rooms in those days and, as she laughingly recalled, the seven-patient ward was often blue with smoke.

Discussing the tight quarters, Kay Brink, who started at McKennan in 1968 and has been with the hospital for 42 years, spoke of patients in the hallways with curtains around them to provide "privacy"—though the curtains did not stop Brink from administering more than a few enemas right there in the hallway.[136] Sister Colman Coakley remembers the constant overcrowding that plagued the hospital throughout the 1950s and well into the 1960s. McKennan placed patients in beds in the hallways, though Sister Colman also wryly noted that Sister Borgia Fitzgerald was a "prime saleswoman" of a bed in the hall: "You'd think she was selling them a suite in the Waldorf!" Because it was the doctors who were most unhappy with the over-crowding, as Sister Colman recollected, they were the ones who spearheaded the effort to expand and modernize the hospital.[137]

New construction was a costly investment as the price tag of medical care and particularly the provision of the latest technology, steadily increased. Nationwide, hospital expenses per patient day more than doubled between the mid-1940s and the mid-1950s, and almost doubled again in the next 10 years.

Average expenses per patient day rose from less than $10 in 1946 to over $44 in 1965.[138]

However, as Margot Nelson, now professor of nursing at Augustana College, remembered: "The men in that room were incredible support for each other. The privacy that we worry about now was, of course, not there. But they razzed each other, they supported each other, they worried about each other, they kept each other company. It really was pretty amazing."[135]

In the early 1950s, for the first time in McKennan's history, the hospital asked the public for financial support in order to expand. As Mother Raphael, then general treasurer of the Presentation Order explained, up to this point the Presentation Sisters had been able to fund hospital expansion on their own but: "because of increased costs and the pressing demand, the problem had become too great."[139]

This first effort at asking the community for money actually came as advice to the hospital from a large group of representative citizens who organized themselves into committees and began to seek donations.[140] As Tom S. Harkison, the general chairman of the Campaign Committee stated: "This need is so glaring and cause so deserving that I believe every thoughtful, civic-minded citizen will be glad to aid generously."[141] Taking the lead to expand the hospital, McKennan's physicians donated some $100,000 toward the $409,506 raised from the community. Led by Dr. S.A. Donahoe, chairman of the doctors' committee, the doctors sought to encourage their colleagues to donate toward much needed improvements. Committee member Dr. P.R. Billingsley emphasized that there were "certain very imperative needs of the institution, primarily more beds." He was seconded by Dr. Pierce McDowell who emphasized that the "situation is becoming very serious."[142] This was put most clearly by Dr. Howard B. Shreves, a member of the doctors' campaign committee, who stated at a community meeting that Sioux Falls population had increased by 10,000 between 1942 and 1952, putting greater pressure on all public facilities and while McKennan had the capacity for approximately 140 adults, "the daily census of beds occupied runs nearer 180."[143] In addition to the money raised by local physicians and the community, the employees of the hospital raised over $13,500 toward the new building.[144]

McKennan also sought federal funding for the new buildings and received a Ford Foundation Grant of $97,100 which was added to a Hill-Burton grant of over $200,000.[145] Congress had passed the Hill-Burton Act in 1946 as a response to the increasing demand for hospital beds as well as a call for a more coordinated plan to provide support for medical care to those areas of the country where facility deficits were greatest. Hill-Burton contributed to an effort to meet national needs. "Between 1946, when the Hill-Burton Act was passed, and 1965, the date of the Medicare legislation, American community hospitals embarked on a new wave of expansion, sustained by the belief in their social utility."[146] In 1955, McKennan began building a new five-floor $1.5 million wing.

After two years of construction, the grand opening came in October of 1957. The new structure, originally planned as a separate building, was later designed to be a connected L-shaped building. The hospital expanded its existing facilities and increased its bed capacity by 65; it also provided new patient services including "routine admission, chest X-rays, premature nursery, dental operating room, fathers' lounge in obstetrics, outpatient department, piped-in oxygen, sun-rooms on every floor, air-conditioning, fire alert alarm system, direct telephone to fire and police departments, audio-intercommunication system and neurological radiography."[147]

The Sisters had welcomed the community's advice regarding the 1955 expansion and, as federal standards and health care became more complicated and running the hospital became more complex, these women continued to welcome the counsel of local business leaders.[148] In 1956, the Board of Trustees, which consisted of Mother Viator Burns and Sisters Borgia Fitzgerald, Bonaventure Hoffman, Camillus Shealy, Leonard Fitzgerald and Bernard Quinn, decided to appoint a lay Advisory Board. Its objective was to act in matters "concerning interrelation between the hospital and the population of service areas, assisting the hospital in improvements of services, broadening the charitable character of the hospital and advising concerning problems mutual to the hospital and the community." The hospital announced that Mr. Henry Quinn would be president of the Advisory Board.[149] Yet, in truth, this was only formalizing what was already happening; Mr. Quinn had been offering advice to the Sisters long before he became president of the Advisory Board. Sister Colman Coakley recollected that Quinn, director of John Morrell & Co. in Sioux Falls, "[came] out and [told] us that we should make some changes with the times…and said that no one in Sioux Falls is paying their employees only once a month, that we should go to every two weeks. That's when we changed."[150]

In addition to the increasing costs and rising complexities of medical care, hospitals also grappled with the challenge that most Americans did not have medical insurance. Throughout the early 20th century, presidents and politicians alike wrestled with the need to bring health insurance to the general populace; a platform that Theodore Roosevelt had advocated in the early part of the century but one that had encountered insurmountable resistance. Franklin Roosevelt was unable to push medical insurance through with the New Deal, and Harry Truman unsuccessfully tried to bring about compulsory health coverage. Nevertheless, while most Americans paid for their care when they saw a doctor, there was a small but growing number who either voluntarily invested in

health insurance or received health insurance through their employer—as industries sought to attract workers by offering them medical benefits. *The New York Times* reported that by 1938, 1 million people had enrolled in hospital insurance and it predicted that the number would be close to 10 million by 1942. Americans who could afford it steadily invested in personal health care insurance and by the 1950s nearly half of the country was enrolled while, by 1960, 122.5 million were part of a voluntary health insurance plan. Nevertheless, the politicians continued to wrangle with the details for a national program.[151]

In 1965, Congress passed Medicare Parts A and B and ushered in dramatic changes. As President Johnson signed the bill he stated: "No longer will older Americans be denied the healing miracle of modern medicine. No longer will illness crush and destroy the savings that they have so carefully put away over a lifetime so that they might enjoy dignity in their later years."[152] Medicare provided persons age 65 and older with medical and hospital benefits; the disabled were folded into the program in 1972. At the same time, Congress also passed Medicaid—a program aimed at persons who did not have the means to pay for health care costs. The entire program was controversial because it brought government into a private industry, and while it provided the elderly with medical care, it also gave hospitals "a license to spend. The more expenditures they incurred, the more income they received." While Medicare was passed with the written expectation that there should be no federal interference in the practice of medicine, with a program of this magnitude, it had to play a role.[153]

A Changing World...

WHILE THE 1960s HAD BROUGHT DRAMATIC CHANGES TO HEALTH CARE, THESE YEARS ALSO DELIVERED A REVOLUTION TO THE LIVES OF THOSE WHO HAD DEDICATED THEMSELVES TO SERVING THE CHURCH AND SOCIETY.

In 1962, the Second Ecumenical Council of the Vatican, or Vatican II, began. While it had an impressive impact on Catholics generally, religious orders were dramatically changed. For the Catholic Sisters of the United States, the modernizing effort by the church challenged their very existence. In the years following Vatican II, women's religious orders underwent a serious self-examination by the church and this led to growing internal divisions within orders. There were those who sought to maintain traditional ways of life, while others embraced the "loosening" of religious rules and regulations. As one young Sister stated—and she may have represented the feelings of many: "We were ambivalent, confused and resentful."[154] At the same time, greater educational and career opportunities for all women diminished the numbers who chose to enter the convent. In the U.S. between 1958 and 1962, female religious orders attracted over 23,000 new members, and in 1965 there were almost 180,000 Roman Catholic Sisters throughout the United States, more than ever before. However, by 1976 only little more than 2,700 women were entering the convent—a drop of 91 percent. In addition, the women who remained were aging and by the early 1990s the average age was 66.[155] Nevertheless, the presence of religious orders continues to be strong in the health care industry, with four of the nation's largest hospital systems being Catholic with combined net revenue of over $18.7 billion.[156]

The Presentation Order of Aberdeen also watched its numbers diminish and membership fell from a high of 503 in 1979 to 155 by 1989; in 2010 the congregation numbered 99 with the average age being 77. Not surprisingly, these changes were also played out at McKennan Hospital as the number of Sisters working on the floors shrank from a high of 28 in 1941 to four in 1991. Mary Clare Julson, McKennan employee and a 1948 graduate of McKennan's School of Nursing reflected on the loss of the Sisters on the floors noting that she felt it was a very big change for the hospital: "They were very conscious of employees. They cared about your future." Julson said the Sisters had a strong influence on the nursing students. "We thought Sister Berchmans Foley had a straight line to heaven. Whenever we needed anything we would go to her."[157] Faced with diminishing numbers in their community, the Presentation Sisters gradually moved to roles in administration and pastoral ministry, rather than providing clinical care. Today the Sisters of the Benedictine and Presentation Orders can be found in Avera McKennan's administration, on its board and on the board of Avera Health. Nevertheless, for all religious orders, as their numbers diminished they increasingly turned the running of their hospitals over to lay persons.

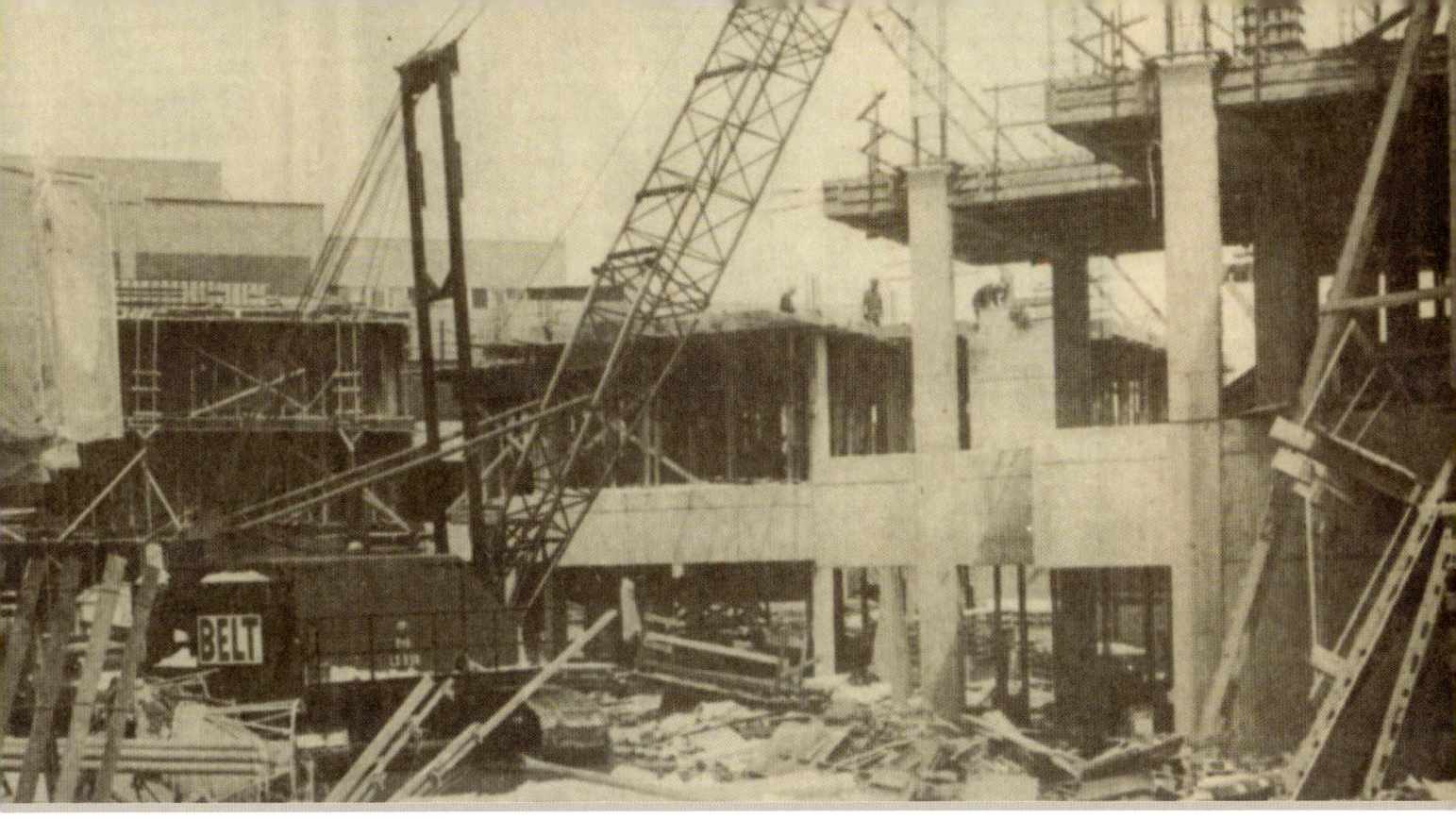

...And Changing Leadership

DURING THE 1960s, ONLY 3 PERCENT OF ADMINISTRATORS IN U.S. CATHOLIC HOSPITALS WERE LAY PERSONS, HOWEVER, BY 1976, 40 PERCENT OF THE 700 CATHOLIC HOSPITALS IN THE UNITED STATES HAD LAY ADMINISTRATORS.

At McKennan, Jim Ward was among the first laymen to take a leadership role, and beginning in 1966 as assistant administrator, Ward played an integral role in the hospital's structural changes for the next 30 years. While he was in charge of nearly half of the hospital's departments, in particular Ward was involved with construction of the buildings for which the hospital was in desperate need: "we had patients in the corridors, sleeping in beds, at that time, behind screens."[158]

As building projects got underway, Ward noted that what made McKennan's construction of the 1970s significant was the establishment of private rooms, "a radical departure from what hospitals had been

doing during that period of time."[159] McKennan's newer areas hosted single, private rooms, the result of the growing evidence that patients heal more quickly when alone and able to rest. McKennan's new administrator, Henry J. Morris, emphasized that these architectural designs provided "optimal individual care."[160]

In July 1970, Morris arrived from St. Joseph Mercy Hospital in Ann Arbor to lead McKennan Hospital. When Morris took the reins, he spent little time dwelling on his status as the first lay administrator at McKennan and, instead, as Morris recollected: "Shortly after arriving, in August, I faced my first crisis…we had to borrow money to meet payroll."

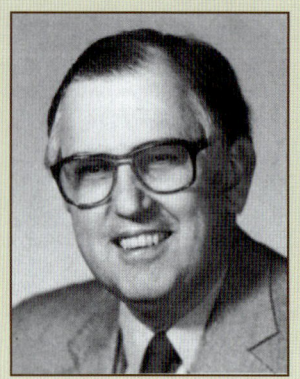

Jim Ward

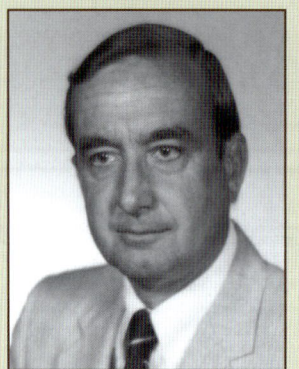

Henry Morris

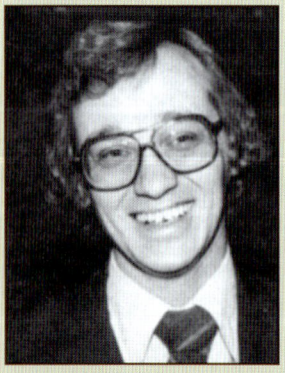

Roger Paavola

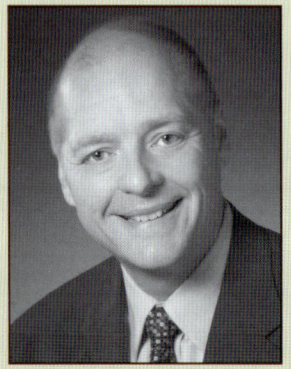

Fred Slunecka

While these economic challenges were the result of a downturn in the U.S. economy, lingering confusion regarding the implementation of Medicare also contributed. Morris sought to steer the hospital through these trials, as medical facilities throughout the country adjusted to changes brought by Medicare. He quickly found his way, and soon joined other U.S. hospitals in borrowing federally supported tax-exempt bonds to pay for needed hospital construction.[161]

In 1973, Sister Colman Coakley, then chair of the McKennan Hospital Board of Trustees, announced McKennan Hospital would add another 240 beds. Sister Colman spoke of this new addition being part of a larger expansion project that had resulted from an outside evaluation of the medical needs of Sioux Falls. This study was clearly reflecting the broader trends in the U.S. for which Medicare now played an important role. "The availability of Medicare reimbursement accelerated the preexisting trends toward borrowing funds for hospital capital projects and deemphasized the role of government grants and private gifts as the basis of funding for new buildings."[162] As a result of governmental spending, by the late 1960s and early 1970s it seemed that society expected hospitals, even non-profits such as McKennan, to upgrade and improve the quality of conditions and patient care.

Completed in the fall of 1975, the new addition raised the hospital's capacity to 356. In 2009, Fred Slunecka, Avera Health chief operating officer and former Avera McKennan regional president, reflected on the significance of the project for the hospital and stated that it was both an impressive financial and a design risk for McKennan to make.[163]

"By today's standards we would just be amazed at the size of that project compared to the operating budget of the time," he commented. Of McKennan's decision to design only private rooms, Slunecka stated: "That was virtually unheard of. To this day…only 30 percent of all hospital beds in America are private rooms, and McKennan Hospital in 1976 was 100 percent private rooms. That's an extraordinary accomplishment for the time."[164]

Challenging Days

DEMAND CONTINUED TO ESCALATE; IN LATE 1980 AND EARLY 1981, THE *ARGUS LEADER* EMPHASIZED THAT MCKENNAN AND SIOUX VALLEY HOSPITALS "WERE FILLED TO OVERFLOWING IN SOME UNITS."

Clearly this situation had been plaguing both institutions for months; as the *Argus Leader* discussed in November of 1980, "a shortage of beds forced administrators…to admit only critically ill patients and to reassess building programs."[165] Not long after this article appeared, McKennan announced that it would add almost 160,000 square feet; hospital capacity grew to 407.[166] Within three months of the March announcement, the hospital broke ground and completed this phase in 1983.

Yet, changes and challenges were brewing for all U.S. hospitals as medical costs escalated despite government efforts to control spending. In 1983, President Ronald Reagan signed legislation altering the government's role in health care payments and Congress quickly passed the legislation into law. "Instead of reimbursing hospitals on the basis of the costs incurred, Medicare was now to pay a set fee per case, with the fee varying by type of diagnosis, for convenience, [diagnoses were] arranged in 467 diagnosis-related groups (DRGs)." This was part of the continued effort at standardization, and sought to put each hospital on a level playing field—with the presumption that they were all run as "businesses in a competitive industry." It also standardized diagnoses which, at minimum, threatened the autonomy of the physician. More importantly, "patient care could be seen—for Medicare, at least—in terms of standardized 'products,'

reinforcing the image of the hospital as a factory."[167] The presumption was that all patients experienced illness in a similar manner and the efficient hospital could take care of the patient during the time frame that the DRG allotted while the inefficient hospital would take longer. Ultimately, those hospitals that failed to "heal" the patient during the given time frame were nevertheless held responsible for the extra costs. Carol DeSchepper, who started her nursing career at McKennan in 1970, remembers the arrival of the DRG and described that it was like having the government hand the hospital a check and directing, "Here, care for your patient with this amount of money." At minimum, recalls DeSchepper, now vice president for quality with Avera Health, this contributed to a reduction of the length of time patients remained in the hospital.[168]

The changes to Medicare were complex with wide-ranging impact as hospitals were expected to act like businesses and offer the best care at the best prices. Similar to for-profit hospitals, non-profit hospitals were undergoing impressive changes between the late 1960s and 1980s. Increasingly, these non-profits went into debt when building new structures, financing building through tax exempt bonds. They were becoming more like their for-profit competitors and, in addition, by the 1980s, were also beginning to market their services.[169] While prior to the mid-1980s, the American Hospital

Association saw advertising as unethical and the American Medical Association refused to allow members to advertise, now marketing was seen as part of doing business.[170]

This new marketing effort was part and parcel of the growing competitive nature of health care and locally the impact of all health care changes became quickly apparent. McKennan and Sioux Valley hospitals struggled; both saw a drop in patients as well as income and, as a result, laid off employees. The *Argus Leader* sought out administrators from both hospitals for comment and McKennan's Roger Paavola and Sister Colman along with Sioux Valley's Lyle Schroeder and Richard Viehwig discussed the changing world of health care. They all agreed that the government had determined that better technology, wellness

programs and an increased expectation for patients to pay for care contributed to the government's decision-making. "Economics, not social responsibility has become the government's primary concern with health care. Insurance companies, businesses who buy group insurance and consumers—who now are asked to help share in hospital costs—also increasingly are asking how much does it cost before they walk through the hospital door." All interviewed recognized that hospitals needed to adapt to the times and used the example of the rise in outpatient surgery to show how technology had transformed the world of medicine.[171]

McKennan particularly faced trying times. In March of 1983, the *Argus Leader* discussed the fact that McKennan had too few patients; between 1980-83 its occupancy rate had dropped from 84 to 77 percent.

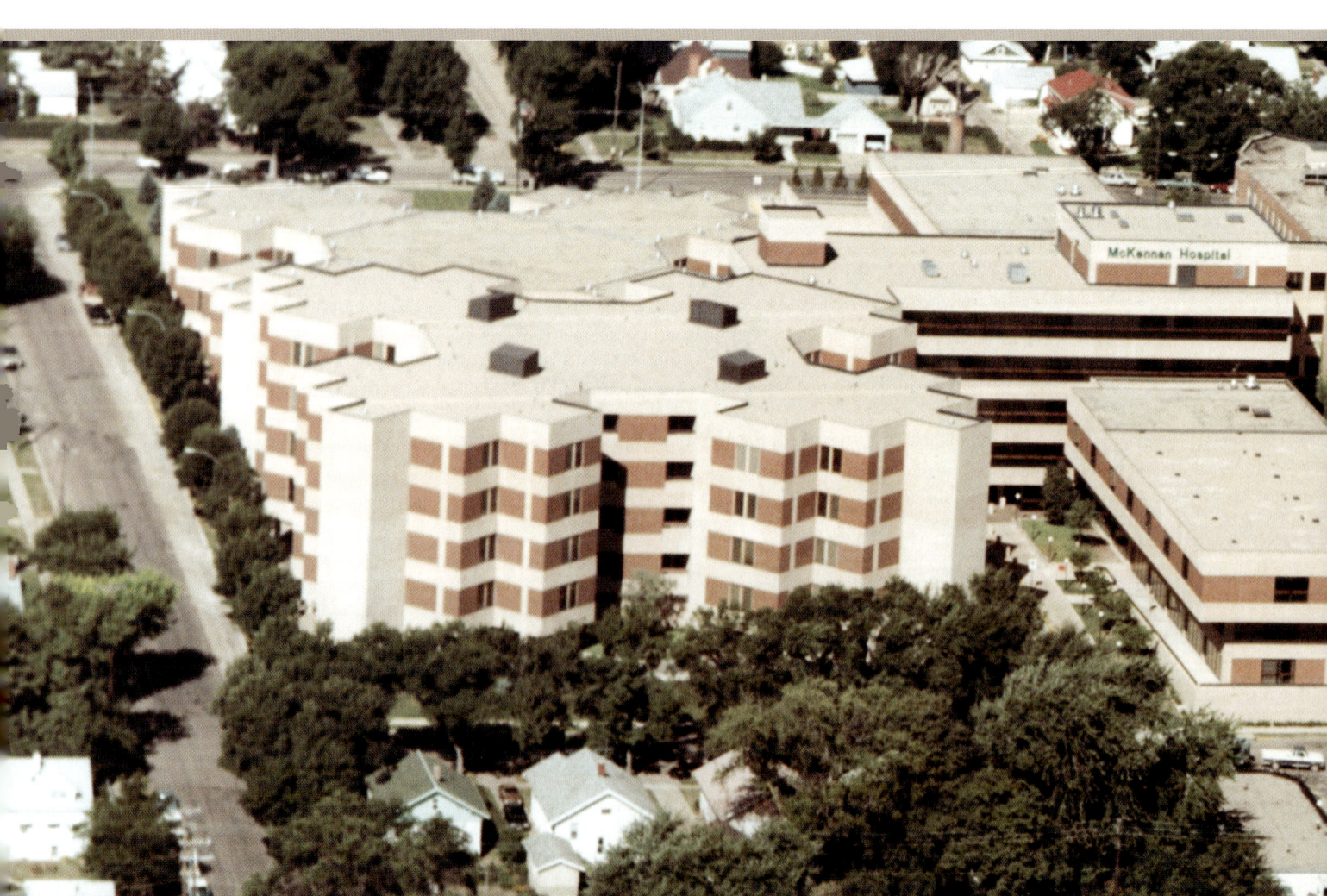

Henry Morris attributed the drop to shorter stays, more specialization and growing financial pressures on patients.[172] McKennan was deeply in debt due to recent expansion, cuts in federal reimbursement and a drop in patient numbers and in 1983, Morris laid off 31 employees, reduced the work hours of 107 and eliminated 59 vacant positions. In December of that year, after 13 years at McKennan Hospital, Henry Morris resigned and Roger Paavola, McKennan's associate administrator, took his place.[173] Nevertheless, circumstances worsened as the hospital's occupancy rate dropped to 60 percent.[174] McKennan's problems were the result of both internal and external challenges.[175]

One impediment for McKennan was that it had been blocked from developing neonatal and heart care services as a result of the 1974 National Health Planning and Resource Development Act that required states to institute what became known as a Certificate of Need. The Certificate of Need (CON) program obligated that each state government approve hospital capital expenditures. The program's intention was to control hospital costs by avoiding duplication, but the result was to allow one hospital to gain a clear competitive advantage over another. This became obvious as Sioux Valley Hospital entered into neonatal and cardiac care in the late 1970s and its patient numbers increased—while McKennan, which dominated in mental health and orthopedic care, was not allowed to offer the more profitable and vital heart and neonatal care services. As a result, McKennan watched its numbers decline.[176] McKennan Hospital needed to apply for Certificates of Need in order to open neonatal intensive and cardiac care units.

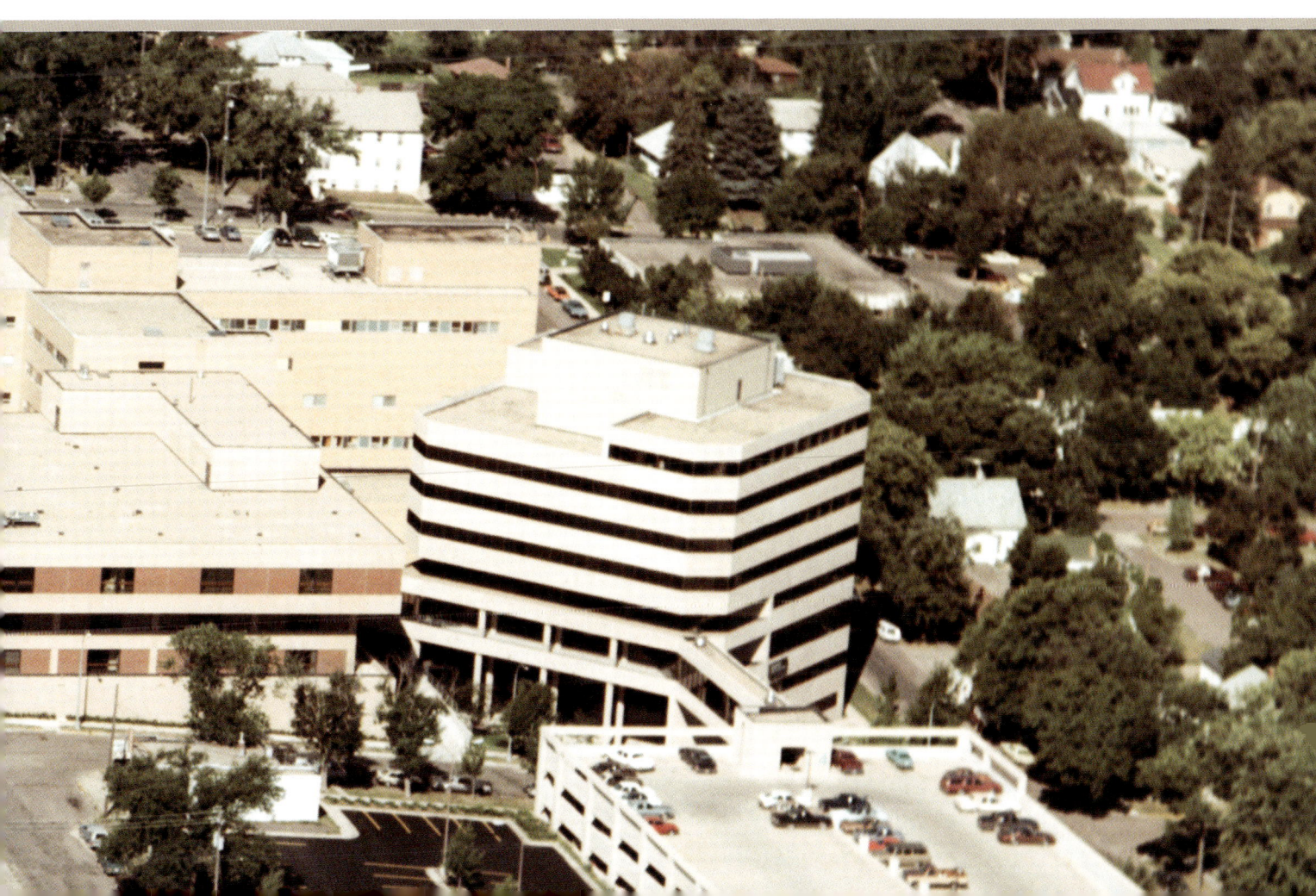

The Future Brightens

By 1988 McKennan had a cardiac care program.

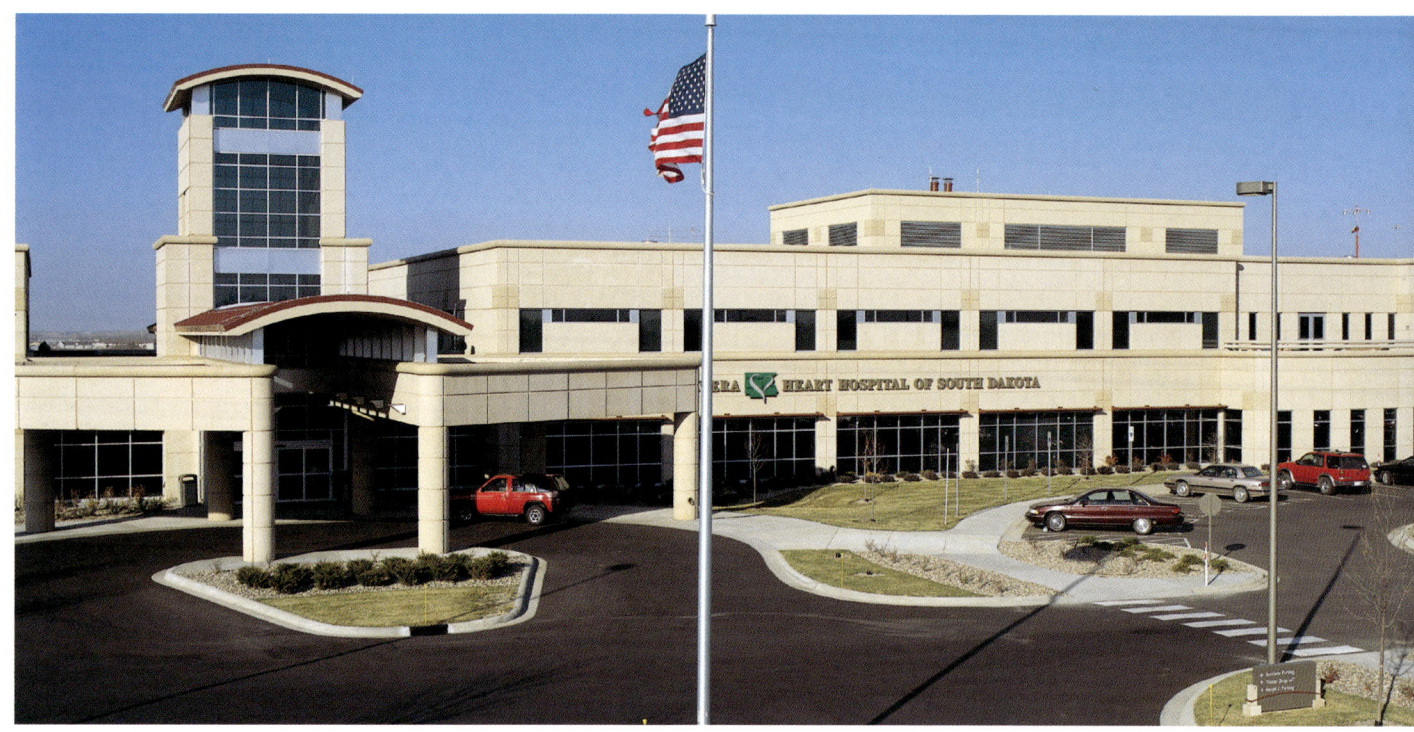

By the mid-1980s, Sioux Valley's North Central Heart Institute (NCH) had two heart catheterization labs and three coronary operating rooms; McKennan decided it was time to make an argument that there was enough demand to enable the region to host another heart program. In 1986, McKennan Hospital applied to the state of South Dakota for a Certificate of Need. Sioux Valley disagreed and its Chief Operating Officer, Jon Soderholm, argued against McKennan's case in a tense fight that erupted over heart care in Sioux Falls. Sioux Valley had profited greatly from its heart program and it opposed McKennan's request for a Certificate of Need. In December, the state ruled in McKennan's favor and granted the hospital's application to offer heart catheterization and open heart surgery. By 1988 McKennan had a cardiac care program.[177] As a result of being able to offer heart surgery among other medical care services, by the early 1990s, impressive changes occurred at McKennan and hospital admissions grew by eight percent each year in both 1991 and 1992.[178]

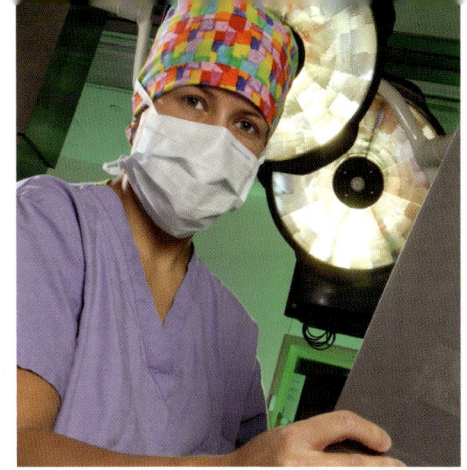

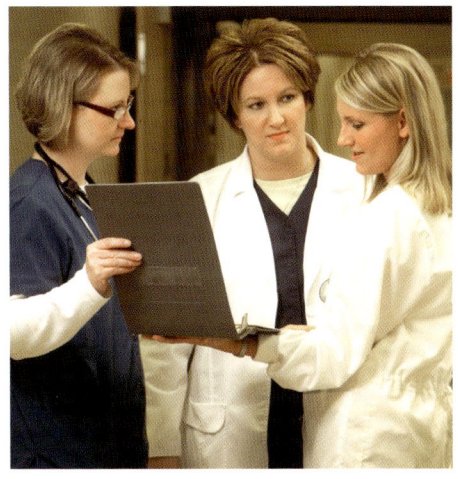

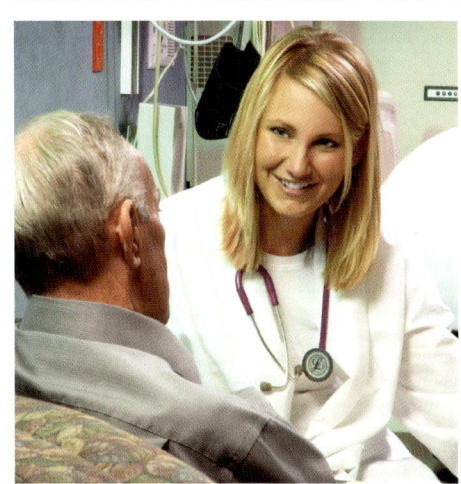

However, by the mid-1990s, there was a surprising turn of events as the doctors of North Central Heart Institute began to feel stifled by the "bureaucracy of large hospitals" and publicly considered leaving Sioux Valley. The heart physicians wanted to establish their own hospital where they felt that, because they could focus solely on heart care and not have the layers of administration required by larger operations, they could be more efficient and thus less costly. This proposal was also about profits going directly to physicians who had watched their incomes drop both as a result of changes to Medicare as well as controls installed under managed care.[179]

In 1998, after receiving financial backing, the physicians of North Central Heart established a partnership with MedCath, a corporation that was building specialty heart hospitals across the country.

McKennan Hospital joined the project arguing that not to do so would undermine McKennan's 10 years in the heart business.[180] McKennan's trustees were also convinced that, if they did not partner with North Central Heart, the community would likely end up with three competing heart programs—one at NCH, one at Sioux Valley Hospital (which had refused to partner with NCH), and one at McKennan. In 1999 construction began on what, at that time, was the largest single building project in Sioux Falls history and the Avera Heart Hospital opened in 2001.

Ironically, the man who would be running the new facility was the same person who had in 1986 argued against McKennan's entrance into heart care: Jon Soderholm. Soderholm, who had been with Sioux Valley Hospital for 31 years and thinks fondly of his time there, had retired from Sioux Valley in 1997.

However, Soderholm was still interested in being part of a medical organization, and as the Heart Hospital was becoming a reality, McKennan approached Soderholm to lead it. As he hired employees for the new entity, Soderholm insisted that physicians and employees agree with his vision for the new hospital. "During the interview process, we talked about the Heart Hospital's values, and if those values were not something they could live with, then I told them don't bother applying."[182] Clearly Soderholm found the right team as the Avera Heart Hospital has been named among 100 Top Hospitals® for cardiovascular care in the country by Thomson Reuters in 2006, 2007, 2008 and 2009.[183]

In 2010, Jon Soderholm must have felt a sense of deja vu when that year's federal health reform bill limited the expansion of physician-owned hospitals. Soderholm, who in 1986, as an employee of Sioux Valley Hospital, had argued against the need for cardiac services at McKennan Hospital, was now arguing against Sanford* Health's expansion of its heart program. Soderholm suggested that there was no need for another large heart facility in Sioux Falls, particularly as heart attack numbers were decreasing with improving preventive measures and the demand for heart surgery was dropping. Nevertheless, Soderholm suggested that he felt, for the near term,

the Avera Heart Hospital would be just fine, but he did express concern that if there was a dramatic change to technology, "it would be problematic for us."[184]

In September of 2010 Avera McKennan purchased MedCath's interest in the Avera Heart Hospital and Avera Heart became a partnership between Avera McKennan and the North Central Heart Institute. As Fred Slunecka wrote when he announced the purchase, "As the only regional hospital dedicated solely to heart and vascular care, we are very proud of the Avera Heart Hospital, and the excellent care it provides. It is the region's first Nationally Accredited Chest Pain Center, and has been on the list of 100 Top Hospitals® for cardiovascular care for the past four years! It remains a very important component of the comprehensive care offered by Avera and we are excited to expand our relationship."[185]

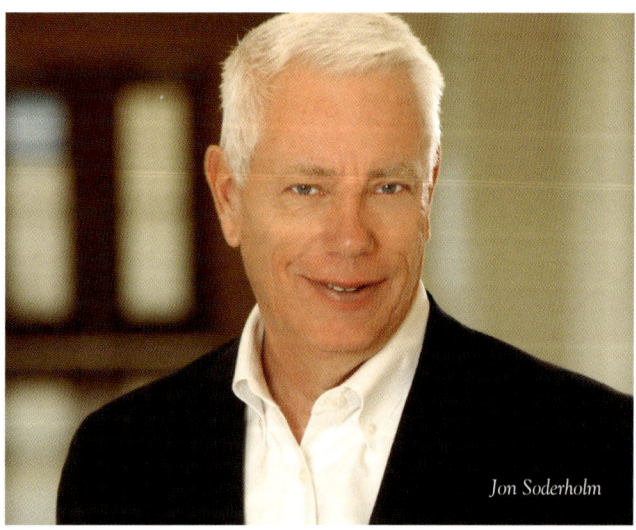

Jon Soderholm

Avera Heart Hospital has been named among 100 Top Hospitals® for cardiovascular care in the country by Thomson Reuters in 2006, 2007, 2008 and 2009.

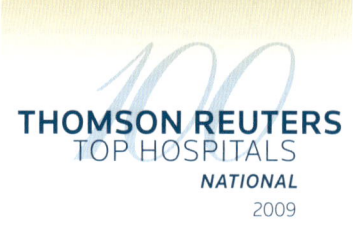

THOMSON REUTERS
TOP HOSPITALS
NATIONAL
2009

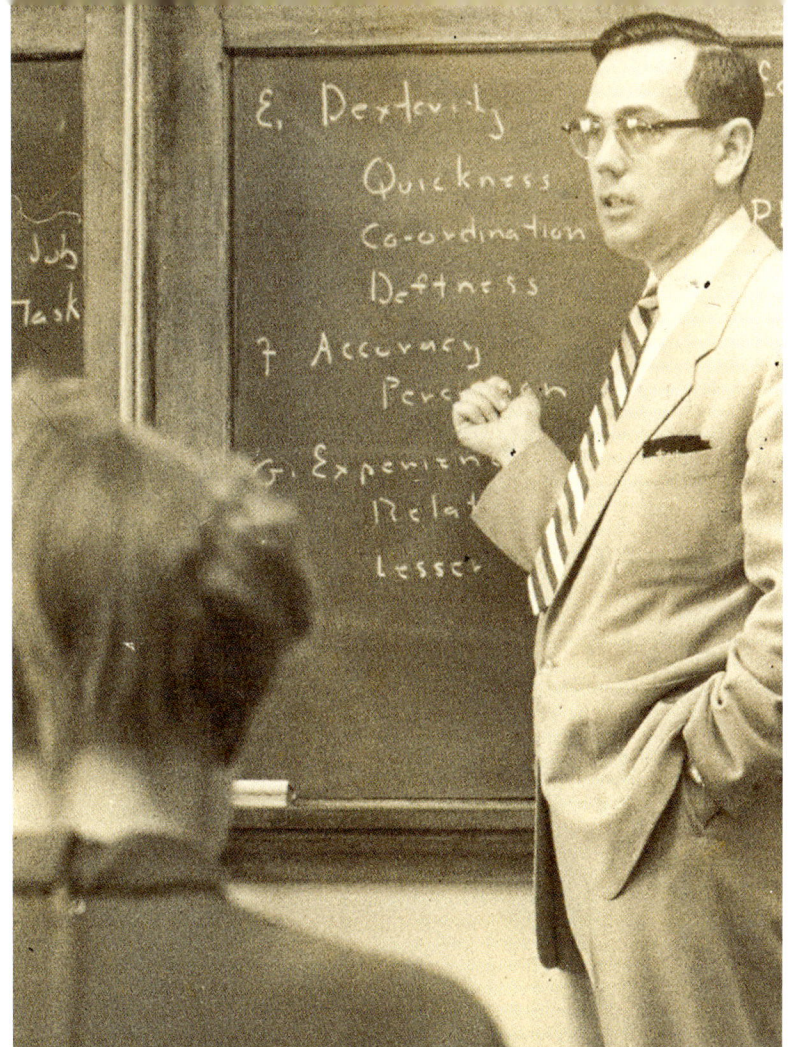

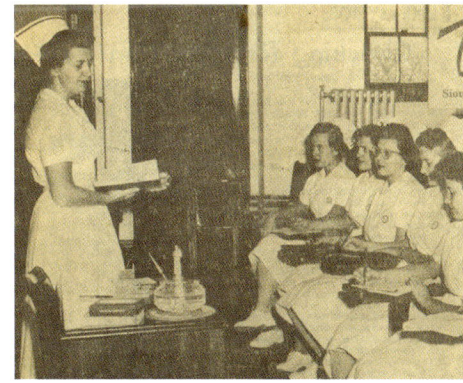

Throughout the century as medicine evolved, South Dakota's need for trained physicians increased and this had a significant impact upon the state's only medical school. The South Dakota School of Medicine, founded in 1907, has its own important history that includes times of triumph and challenge. One of the more challenging stages for the school was in the early 1970s, when it struggled financially; so perilous were its circumstances that it had trouble meeting payroll.[186] A major hurdle was that it was only a two-year program and while nearly 100 percent of the students went on to a four-year degree, only 18 percent returned to South Dakota to practice. In addition, by 1974, South Dakota had fallen to 50th in the nation regarding physician-to-patient ratio.[187] Thus, the school either needed to close or to expand its program from two to four years and there was a growing call for the school to move to a four-year model.

Educating Future Medical Personnel

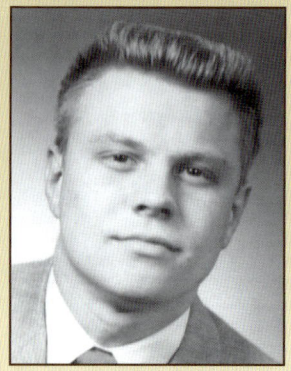

Dr. Loren Amundson

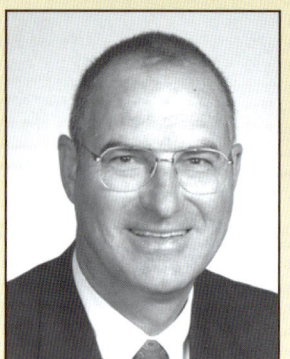

Dr. Al Hartmann

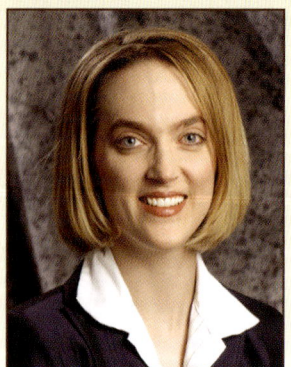

Dr. Jennifer McKay

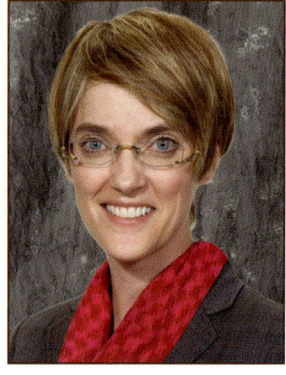

Dr. Kimberlee McKay

As McKennan administrator, Henry Morris, reflected on his tenure at the hospital, he noted that one of his priorities was to bring more physicians into South Dakota. Morris felt that one way to do this was to have a four-year medical school in South Dakota. "We needed to make Sioux Falls, McKennan Hospital and the state of South Dakota more attractive to recruiting physicians." Morris recollected that one challenge was how to provide a hospital setting in which third- and fourth-year medical students could gain experience. The idea was floated that a "school without walls" could be created; in this model, the medical school uses existing hospitals and clinics for training purposes, rather than, as in traditional programs, the medical school owns a hospital in which its students learn the profession.[188]

Over the next few years, the South Dakota School of Medicine worked to create a curriculum, hire faculty and develop relationships with local hospitals. McKennan, Veterans and Sioux Valley hospitals of Sioux Falls and Sacred Heart Hospital of Yankton all signed contracts to be part of the program; the plan was for each to play a role as a teaching hospital for the school.[189] "The first junior class began class May 12, 1975, with 27 assigned to Sioux Falls and 13 to Yankton." The effort was a success; in February of 1977 the school received accreditation for two years and on May 14, 1977, the South Dakota School of Medicine graduated its first class.[190] Nevertheless, there were still many questions and much work to be done as the school particularly struggled with inadequate budgets. Regardless, the hope was that the establishment of a four-year medical school in South Dakota would contribute to an end to South Dakota's physician shortage.[191]

As time progressed, the South Dakota School of Medicine steadily gained more external recognition and longer terms of accreditation; by the late 1980s, the school was on solid footing. Indeed, the school's Yankton-based team curriculum received national acknowledgment as other medical schools, including Harvard University, considered using the Yankton curriculum design as a model. Then, in 1991, the school welcomed a $6 million gift from Sioux Valley Hospital to fund a building to house a branch of the medical school in Sioux Falls—on Sioux Valley's campus.[192]

The South Dakota School of Medicine continued to receive accolades and grant funding. In 2000, Sioux Valley Hospital donated $10 million and was granted permission to use the school's name for the next 30 years. At the same time, Avera McKennan Hospital became Avera McKennan Hospital & University Health Center to reflect the hospital's "leadership role in medical education in the region," and to emphasize the fact that the state medical school was not "owned" by any private donors but was a state institution supported by all taxpayers.[193] In 2006, T. Denny Sanford donated $400 million to Sioux Valley Hospital and the organization changed its name to Sanford Health. In addition, Sanford, through the newly named Sanford Health, donated $20 million to the medical school and university officials agreed to change the school's name to the Sanford School of Medicine of the University of South Dakota. That same year, Avera McKennan committed to funding 14 $12,000 scholarships annually for first- and second-year medical students.[194] As another way to support health sciences at local schools, over a 10-year period beginning in November of 2007, Avera Health donated $15 million to South Dakota State University as the school and hospital entered into a partnership to expand the university's health science and research programs.[195]

Establishing the medical school as a four-year program has proven to be beneficial. As a 2000 graduate and now Avera McKennan hospitalist, Dr. Jennifer McKay, stated in 2010: "I think one could credit the USD School of Medicine for diverting a crisis in health care availability in South Dakota. Now that [they] are a four-year school many of those physicians come back." Just as she and her twin sister, Dr. Kimberlee McKay, Obstetrics/Gynecology specialist at Avera Women's did—and they "felt very good about coming home."[196]

In addition to its connections with the state medical school, McKennan Hospital has long been a site for postgraduate medical training. In the 1950s, McKennan provided a one-year internship for graduates from foreign medical schools; in July of 1964 a more formal internship program was initiated.[197] In 1974, McKennan Hospital and Sioux Valley Hospital contributed funds to start a three-year family practice residency in Sioux Falls. These new medical school graduates gained one year of general training before entering into specialized areas such as ophthalmology, anesthesia or dermatology. The residency's first director was Dr. Lloyd Sweeney; the associate director was Dr. Loren Amundson. McKennan is also host to several "flexible" interns each year.[198]

Dr. Al Hartmann, director of the Medical Education Program at McKennan from 1976 to 2005, noted that the interns and residents gain a quality education at the hospital but they also provide service. In earlier years, they staffed the emergency room and were on hospital premises to offer support in many areas. A more subtle continuing benefit of their presence, Dr. Hartmann said, is that having students and residents around keeps experienced practitioners up-to-date in their fields. "There's no better way to keep current than to teach somebody."[199]

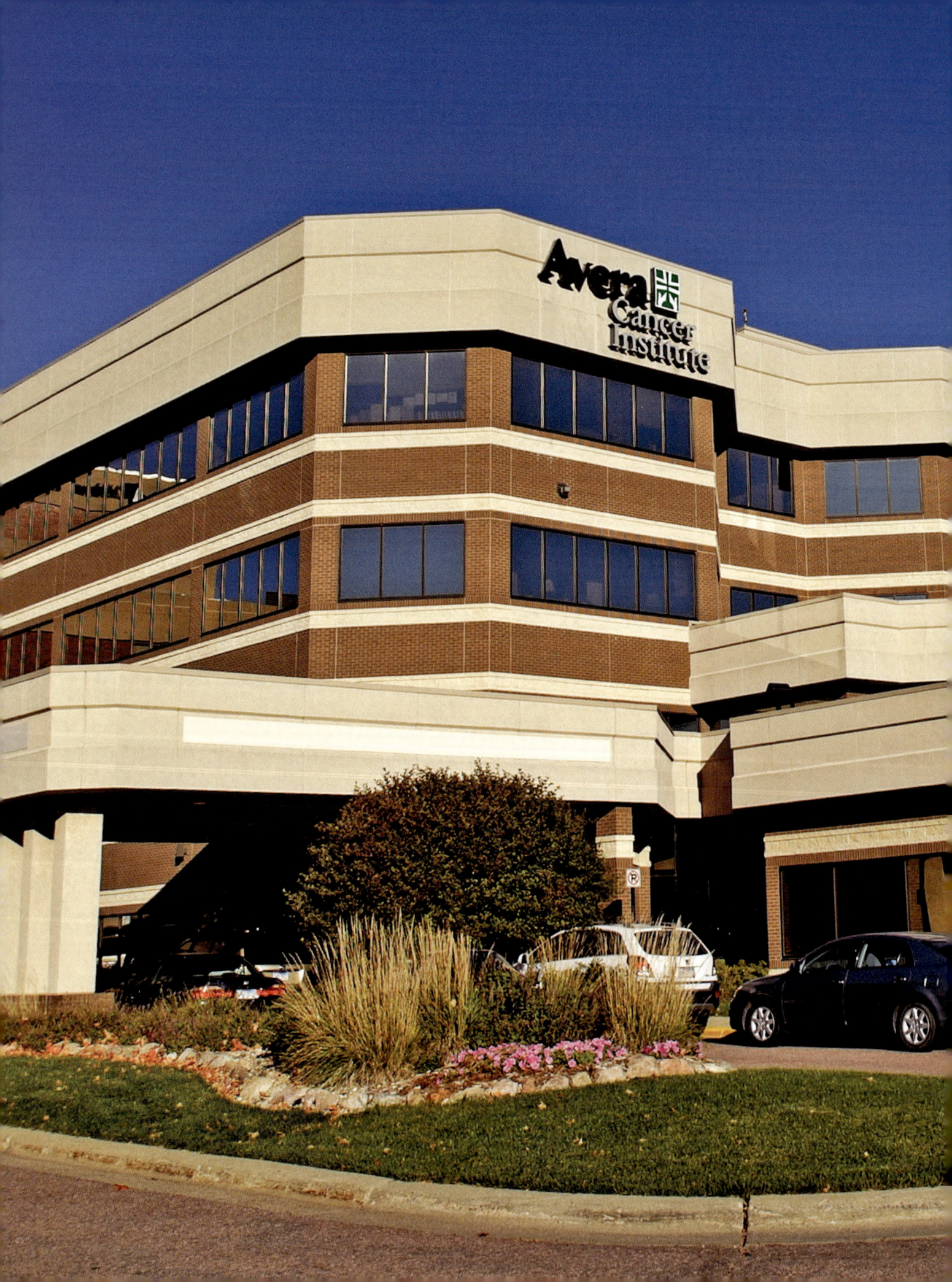

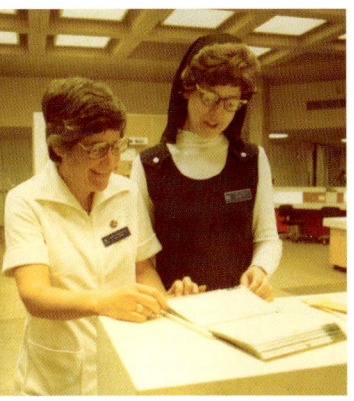 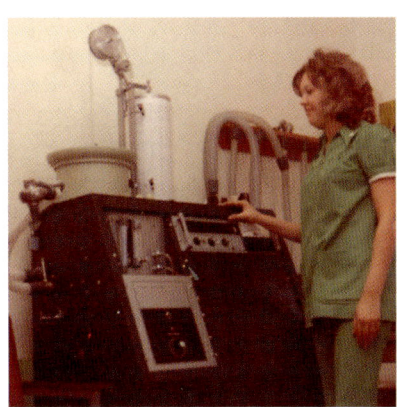 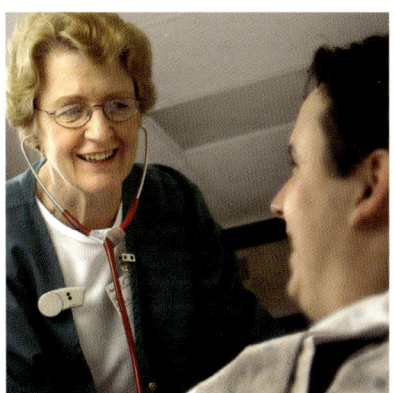 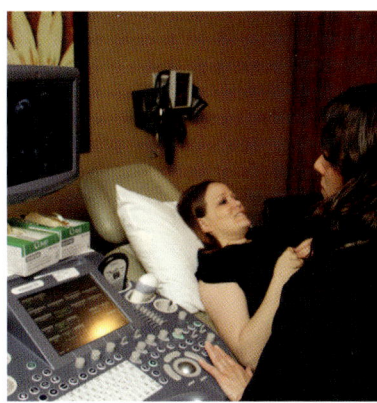

The Rise of Sub-Specialties in Sioux Falls

In 2009, Jon Soderholm spoke of how the establishment of a four-year medical school contributed to making Sioux Falls the setting for specialty medical services.[200]

He reflected on how in the late 1960s and early 1970s medical sub-specialties in Sioux Falls, "changed us from being a sleepy, dusty farm town providing health care to the start of being a community which provided significant specialty care." It also, in Soderholm's recollection, put pressure on the primary care physicians who were in the majority in Sioux Falls because they soon had competition from doctors that specialized in particular areas.[201] Examples of the evolution of medical specialties at McKennan can be observed in the development of cancer care and organ transplant services.

In 1989 McKennan broke ground on a $6.5 million cancer center and in May of 1991 the Dakota Midwest Cancer Institute opened. The hospital invited cancer survivor, activist and actress Ann Jillian to speak at the reception that introduced the 43,000-square-foot building to the public. In little more than 10 years the Avera Cancer Institute had far surpassed expectations and outgrown its facilities.[202]

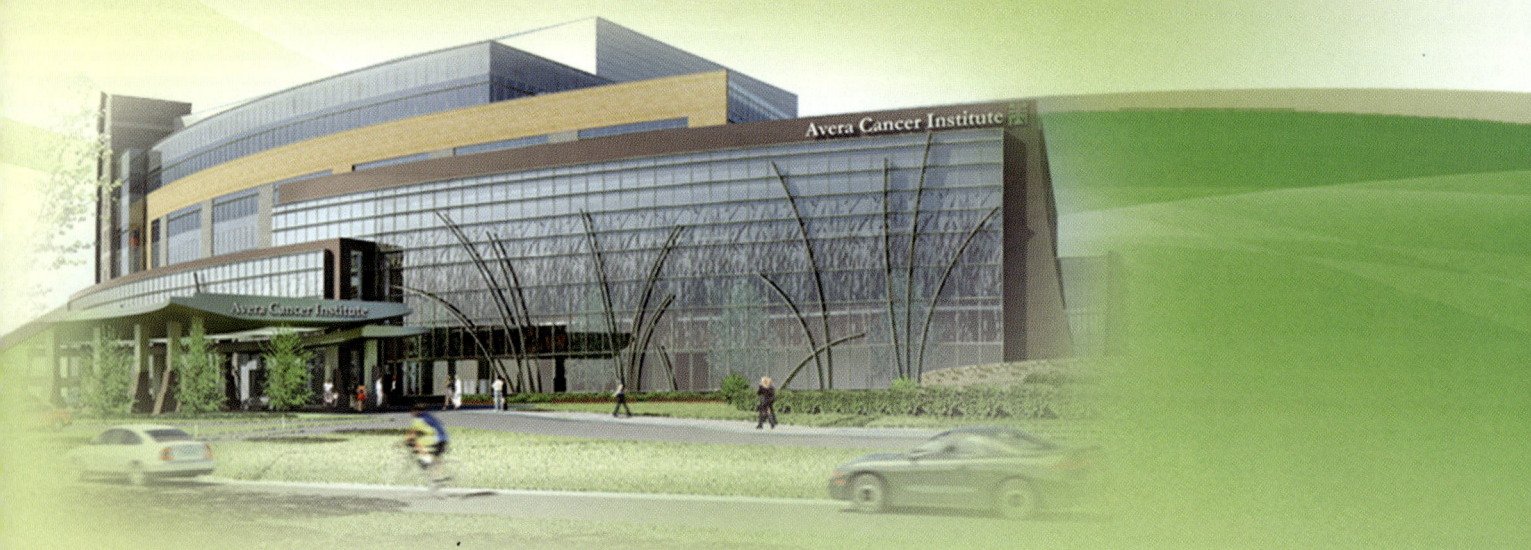

Hence, on May 19, 2008, Avera McKennan broke ground on the new $93 million Avera Cancer Institute that is four times the size of the former building – the largest construction project in Sioux Falls history. "This will place us at the level of world class," stated Fred Slunecka, who toured top cancer centers across the U.S. as designs were developed.[203]

The Prairie Center, home of Avera Cancer Institute and Avera Surgery Center, will also be the first health building "in the state of South Dakota and the wider region" registered as a Leadership in Energy and Environmental Design (LEED) project by the U.S. Green Building Council. The Avera Cancer Institute is also pursuing Green Globe Certification, "the leading worldwide certification based on internationally accepted standards for environmental sustainability."[204] To achieve greater energy efficiency, the building uses natural materials including wood and stone, leaves a great deal of space for plants and greenery, offers natural lighting to reduce the need for artificial light and has an expansive exterior green area with native plantings and a walking trail. In addition to using recycled building materials, the hospital purchased building supplies locally in order to save on transportation costs.[205] "This is going to be one of the most highly advanced, environmentally friendly buildings in the Upper Midwest," stated Richard

Molseed, senior vice president of Environmental Services.[206] He anticipates that these environmentally friendly plans will also contribute to the patient healing process.[207]

Most importantly, the building is here to provide care to those affected by cancer. As oncologist Dr. Addsion Tolentino stated: "My patients will have access to the latest technology under one roof." The Avera Cancer Institute offers care in a variety of specialties including radiation oncology, medical oncology, bone marrow transplant, hematology and gynecologic oncology. As former chief of staff Dr. Patty Peters noted, the Avera Cancer Institute uses the team approach for cancer care; for example, a woman with breast cancer will have her case brought before a team of doctors: "Family docs, surgeons, plastic surgeons, oncologists, radiation oncologists, pathologist, radiologists—they all work together to help a woman through this breast cancer process."[208]

The center hosts over 50 infusion suites for chemotherapy that offer patients a private setting in which they will look out at the gardens and green space of the building so as to enhance "the healing effects of nature" noted Kris Gaster, Avera McKennan's assistant vice president of Outpatient Cancer Clinics.[209] Fred Slunecka discussed all that the new building had to offer and suggested that what made the Avera Cancer Institute special was not just the technology that "fewer than a handful of institutions nationwide have" but also that the building's aesthetics and "the effort to not just work on the physical illnesses but to work as much or more on the spiritual aspects. The healing aspects of care are just as important, obviously, as the technical aspects. We are very committed to the mind-body-spirit of all cancer patients. And that's what makes it unique and special."[210]

In addition to offering some of the latest technology, as a result of a grant of over $2 million provided by The Leona M. and Harry B. Helmsley Charitable Trust, the Avera Surgery Center will conduct research-based treatment.

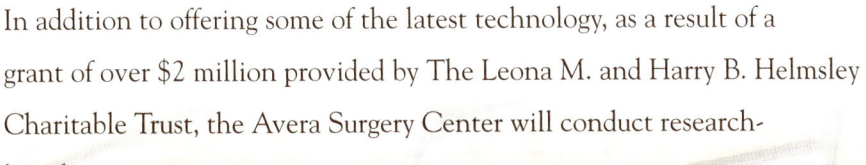

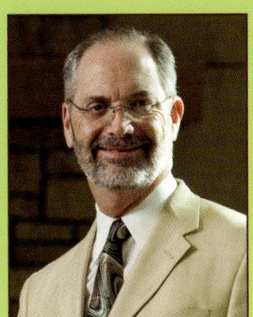

Richard Molseed

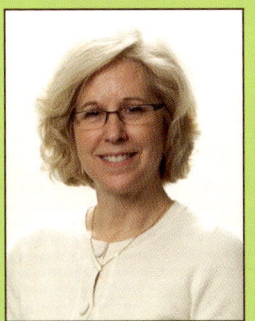

Kris Gaster

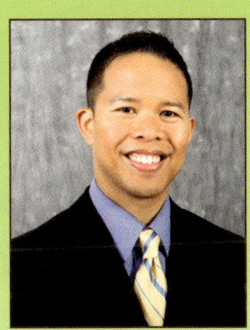

Dr. Addison Tolentino

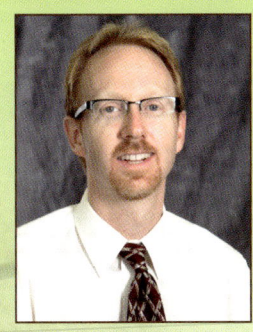

Dr. Kelly McCaul

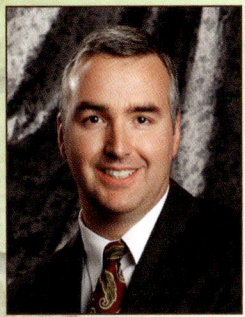

Dr. Wade Dosch

using Intra-operative Radiation Therapy (IORT), which allows surgeons to administer radiation during cancer surgery. This procedure, which is only offered in only 12 other hospitals in the country, enables the physicians to reduce post-operative radiation treatment. It is certainly meant to help those patients for whom traveling for radiation is a hardship. Dr. Wade Dosch, one of two surgeons and three radiation oncologists involved with introducing this surgical procedure, explained the value of the treatment for women with breast cancer who live in rural communities where receiving six weeks of radiation may require temporarily relocating to another town and thus is a great hardship. "It is heartbreaking to watch a woman choose to have a mastectomy because she cannot tolerate the time commitment required of radiation therapy after breast conservation. Offering a treatment that will decrease post-operative radiation visits will help women decide to pursue breast conservation instead of mastectomy," Dr. Dosch said.[214]

As the Avera Cancer Institute and Avera Surgery Center look to a new future, another specialty that Avera McKennan has been involved with for over 10 years is also expanding and developing. In 1992 McKennan applied to the United Network of Organ Sharing for permission to open the state's first kidney transplant program; it hoped to begin with

18 to 20 transplants annually. In 1993, McKennan Hospital hosted the first kidney transplant in the state under the leadership of Dr. John Ryan, chair of surgery at the South Dakota School of Medicine.[215] Traditionally, transplant programs were established in large metropolitan areas, not in cities as small as Sioux Falls, and this made McKennan's entrance into this specialty unique. The hospital next added pancreas and bone marrow transplant programs.

In 1996, McKennan began its bone marrow transplant program—a process that involves harvesting a patient's own stem cells and treating them with high levels of chemotherapy before returning the marrow to the patient. Dr. Kelly McCaul, the program's medical director, who came to Avera McKennan in 2000 noted, "We offer the same technology and expertise as anywhere else with the compassionate, personalized care that characterizes Avera." In 2004 the Foundation for Accreditation of Cellular Therapy accredited Avera McKennan's bone marrow transplant program, an accolade McCaul noted, "that many large-size programs do not have."[216]

Ten years after the state's first kidney transplant, Avera McKennan established a pancreas transplant program—a need which is particularly common for persons with Type-1 diabetes.[217] "The operation is more extensive and carries with it more risk than kidney transplant. Because candidates are chosen very carefully, and there are fewer pancreases

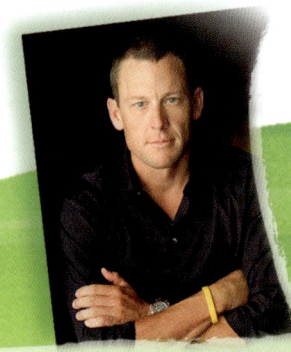

*In October of 2010, Lance Armstrong, Seven-time **Tour de France** winner, cancer survivor and author spoke at the opening of the Avera Cancer Institute.*

available, transplant centers nationally perform fewer pancreas transplants." Avera McKennan has a national reputation for its work and the U.S. Department of Health and Human Services has awarded the Medal of Honor for Organ Donation to the Avera Transplant Institute every year since the award was begun in 2005. In August of 2008, Avera McKennan conducted its 500th solid organ transplant. Avera McKennan's next goal is to begin a liver transplant program. In 2007, the hospital established the Avera Center for Liver Disease and looks forward to conducting its first transplant in the near future.[218]

Avera McKennan has contributed in many other ways to Sioux Falls becoming a city that offers specialized medical care. In addition to cancer care and organ transplant, the hospital offers specialized care in a number of medical needs including dermatology; ear, nose and throat; endocrinology; gastroenterology; hematology; hepatology; infectious disease; internal medicine; neonatology; nephrology; neurology and neurosurgery; obstetrics/gynecology; gynecologic oncology; medical oncology; orthopedics; pediatrics; perinatology; physiatry; interventional radiology; radiation oncology; sports medicine; surgery (including bariatric, plastic and transplantation); urology; and vascular services.

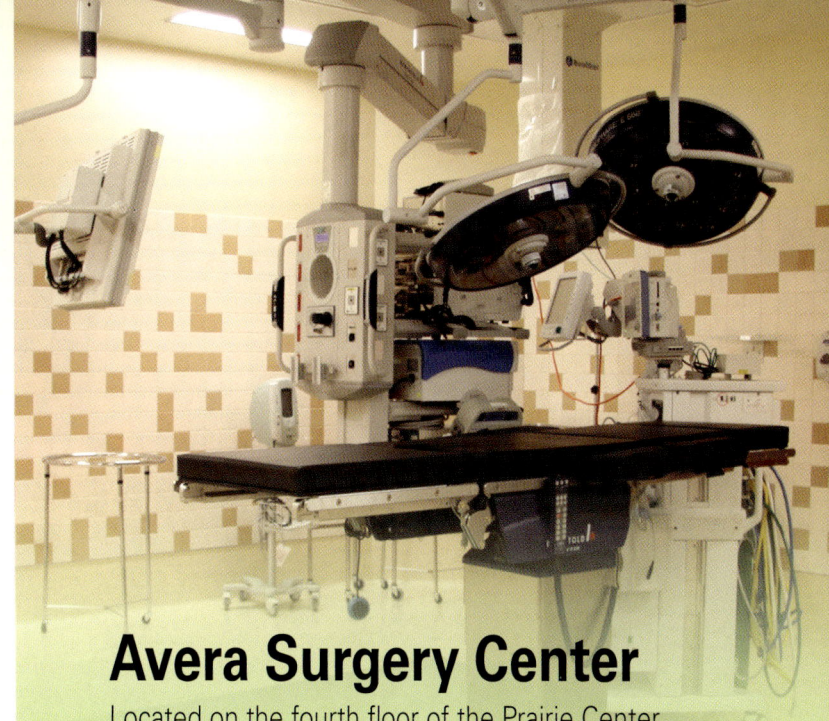

Avera Surgery Center
Located on the fourth floor of the Prairie Center

Fred Slunecka argued Avera McKennan needed a surgery center in order to be more competitive in Sioux Falls' health care market.[211] Opened in July of 2010, the Avera Surgery Center hosts eight surgical suites that are the largest operating rooms in Sioux Falls. "The size of the room accommodates the technology we have today, and is also designed to future proof ourselves for evolving technology that we can't predict at this point," said Dr. Greg Schroeder, medical director of operative services and chief of anesthesia at Avera McKennan.[212]

The surgery center will make it more convenient and efficient for patients who need outpatient procedures because it will not integrate them into the main hospital. In the main hospital, moving outpatient services to the new center opens up surgical suites for more complex cases. "We are a Level II Trauma Center," stated Patti Jagoe, assistant vice president of Perioperative Services, "and as such we need to get trauma patients to surgery immediately in order to save lives."

In order to ensure the most up-to-date facility, Avera physicians and surgeons considered the changing needs of medicine and technology and also traveled to other surgery centers to see the latest designs. The surgery center also offers a separate area for parents with children who need surgery; parents can accompany their child to the OR until after they are placed under anesthesia and can be in the recovery room when the child wakes up.[213]

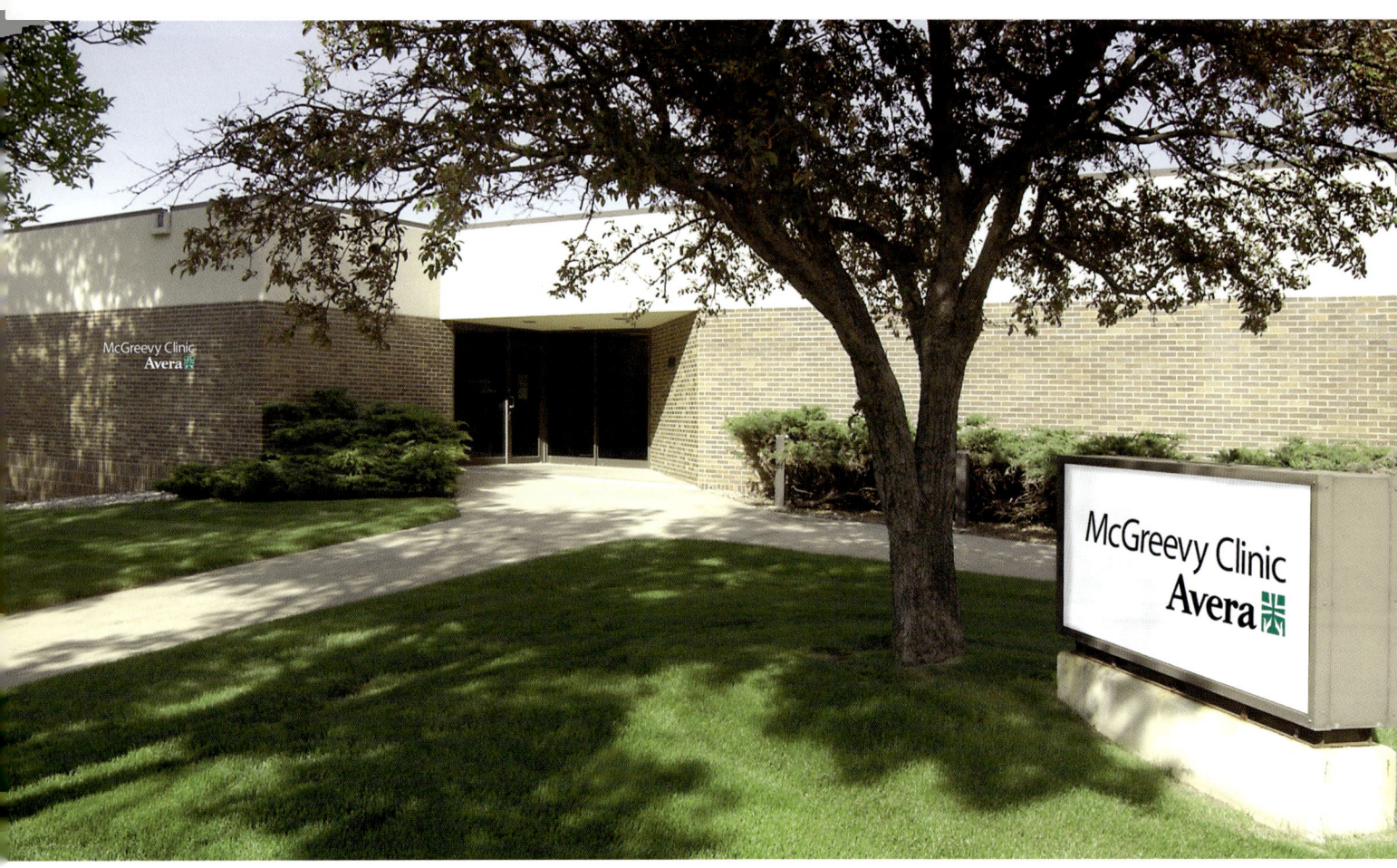

McGreevy Clinic
Avera

From Hospital to Health System

At the same time that Sioux Falls was becoming a center for medical specialties, another nationwide trend was developing in which McKennan Hospital also took part and this was the evolution of hospitals from stand-alone facilities into health systems.[219] During the 1980s, McKennan began the process of affiliating with smaller hospitals and clinics. As a result of the steady growth in managed care and the increasing demands of changing technology, physicians began shifting away from their historical roots in self-employment toward salaried employment. From 1988 to 1996, the share of salaried physicians rose from 28 percent to 48 percent nationally.[220] McKennan Hospital developed a network that integrated doctors

and medical facilities region-wide, and the evolution of creating a much more amalgamated medical system can be seen through McKennan's relationship with McGreevy and Central Plains clinics.

Central Plains Clinic—originally called the Donahoe Clinic—was founded by Drs. S.A. Donahoe and Geoffrey I. Cottam in 1949 and was first located on the ninth floor of the National Bank Building in downtown Sioux Falls. After expansion and relocation, in 1976 the clinic bought 17 acres of land on Kiwanis Avenue and, now with close to 70 physicians on staff, took the new name Central Plains Clinic.[221]

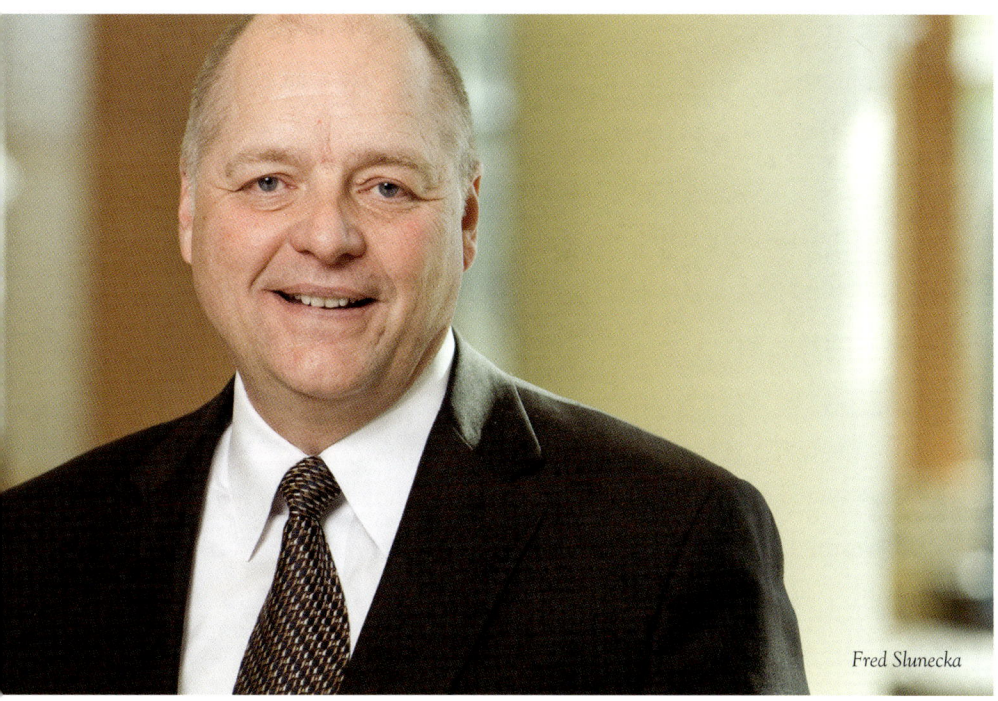

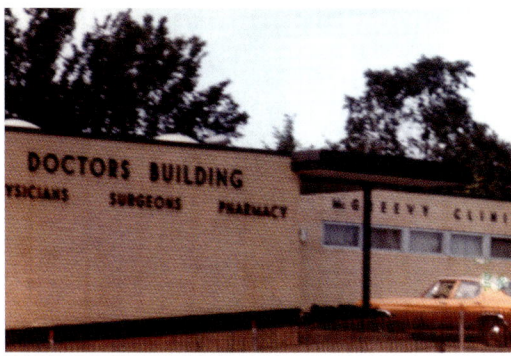

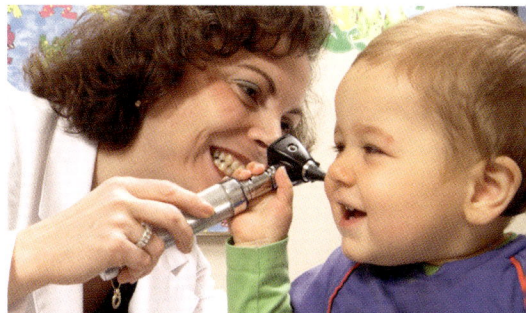

Fred Slunecka

In the early 1990s, the clinic entered into an agreement with McKennan Hospital after Fred Slunecka, Avera Health chief operating officer, suggested to Central Plain's administrator, Edward Arshem, that they move the clinic to the hospital campus. As Slunecka recalled "we laughed and didn't think that was very realistic." However, the joke was on Slunecka as he was soon considering serious possibilities. In January of 1990, the plans began to take shape for Central Plains to move into a new $16 million building on McKennan's campus with the hospital taking over the Central Plains Clinic's Kiwanis site.[222] In 2009 Slunecka reflected on Central Plains Clinic's move:

> *"Clearly one of the biggest points in my career and one of the biggest points in the history of the institution was moving Central Plains Clinic on to the McKennan Hospital campus. That was an extraordinary set of events. It came because of a very close working relationship between myself and the clinic leadership. It came because we were willing to take a chance and to step outside our normal comfort zones to do a very complex real estate deal, to take on a construction project unlike anything we had ever done before as an institution, and so it was big step."[223]*

Yet, the relationship between Avera McKennan and CPC faltered as the clinic began to lose revenue as well as some of its doctors and the relationship between the two organizations became strained. In 2001 Sioux Valley announced plans to buy CPC and Avera McKennan's Slunecka cried foul and stated that the hospital wanted the opportunity to negotiate a deal

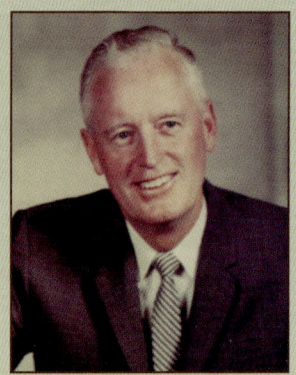

Dr. John McGreevy

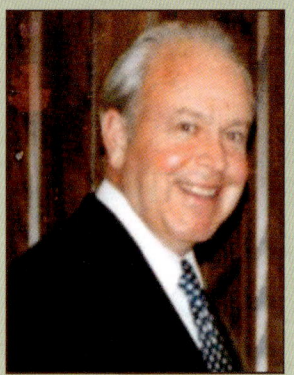

Dr. Ed McGreevy

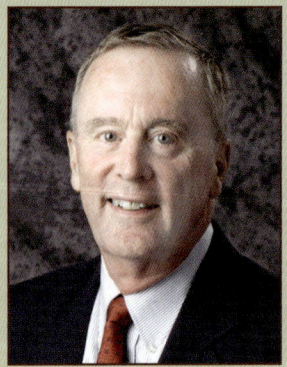

Dr. Pat McGreevy

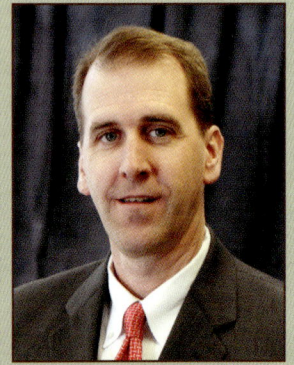

David Flicek

with the clinic. Nevertheless, according to David Danielson, CPC's administrator, McKennan had not been supportive when the clinic's monetary problems became evident. Slunecka countered that this was not the case. The deal between CPC and Sioux Valley moved ahead which led to Sioux Valley employing approximately one-third of Sioux Falls' doctors—a significant blow to Avera McKennan's revenues and position.[224]

As a result of the Central Plains Clinic move, the hospital acknowledged that while it had a good foothold in rural South Dakota, it did not have as strong a position with clinics in Sioux Falls. David Flicek, chief administrative officer of Avera Medical Group, advocated that Avera McKennan needed to gain traction in the primary care market in Sioux Falls. This occurred in 2006 when Avera McKennan purchased McGreevy Clinic.

Dr. John McGreevy established McGreevy Clinic in Sioux Falls when he relocated his practice from Mitchell in 1946. McGreevy originally rented space in the building that housed Moe Hospital on 14th and Main. McGreevy's brother, Dr. Ed McGreevy soon joined the practice. The two men worked at the clinic into the 1960s when they decided to build near McKennan Hospital because John, as his son Dr. Pat McGreevy recalled, was "a big fan of the Presentation Sisters." In the mid-1960s, Drs. Neil Elkjer and Lou Barnett joined the practice; in 1969, Drs. Greg Naughton and Pat McGreevy arrived.

In 1973, McKennan Hospital purchased the McGreevy Clinic building in order to expand, and the practice moved north of the hospital where it remains to the present. Nevertheless, the clinic continued to grow. While in 1980 there were 10 doctors, by 1995 the practice had doubled. In 2007, McGreevy Clinic had over 50 doctors working in various clinics around the city and, as Pat McGreevy noted in an interview, among these are doctors who have come to Sioux Falls from around the globe, including from India, Lebanon, and South Korea.

The son of clinic founder John McGreevy, Dr. Pat McGreevy carried on his father's legacy and further nourished the growth of the clinic. Pat McGreevy grew up in Sioux Falls and fondly remembered being brought to McKennan Hospital when his father did rounds. Pat and his younger brother would sit in the front entrance in the waiting area and, as Pat recalled, there was a Sister in full habit at the front desk. "I don't remember her name…[but] she was very impressive. She admitted patients, served the information desk for visitors, ran the switchboard, answered the phone, made entries into the ledger book all at the same time and with a never-failing friendliness and politeness…this was long before the days of mission statements but she was a mission statement." Pat McGreevy, who received his undergraduate degree from the University of Notre Dame and attended Creighton Medical School, spent 15 years on the Board of Trustees of McKennan Hospital.[225] Throughout his career, McGreevy sought to mentor younger doctors, particularly women, whose numbers at the hospital were slowly increasing.

One young physician that McGreevy mentored was Dr. Patricia Peters. A graduate of Augustana College's nursing program, Peters graduated from medical school at the University of South Dakota in 1980.

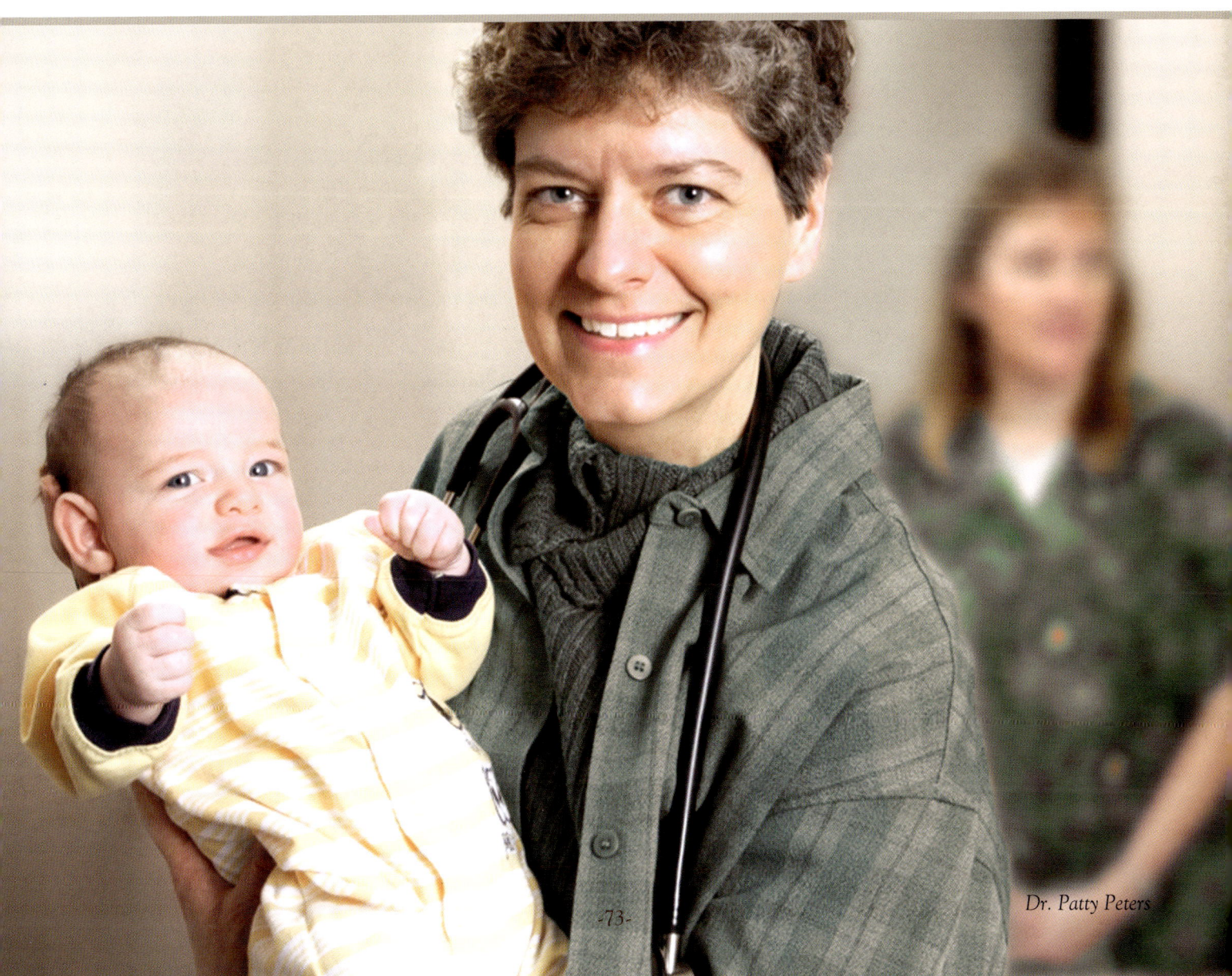

Dr. Patty Peters

When she completed her family practice residency in Sioux Falls in 1983, Peters was invited to practice at McGreevy Clinic by Dr. Ed McGreevy. She was the first woman physician to join the clinic. Pat McGreevy encouraged Peters to become an officer in the hospital's medical staff. She made her way up the ranks from secretary of the family practice department to vice chair of the department. In the early 1990s, Peters became McKennan's chief of staff and after she completed her term in this position, she was invited to be on the Presentation Health System Board of Trustees. After many years of service to the hospital, Peters returned to family practice full time and, "[I] still deliver babies and see young and old."

Peters reflected on the role of clinics in Sioux Falls and their increasingly close relationship with the hospitals. Doctors sought to decide whether to remain independent or work as part of the health system and the challenge was maintaining the clinic's independence and unique nature once under the hospital's umbrella. A number of clinics, including Central Plains Clinic and University Physicians, disintegrated as the physicians either chose to remain with the hospital or move on to establish independent practices elsewhere. Peters also recognized the challenges that every hospital and medical clinic faced: getting patients to come in their doors. The changing environment required clinics to become much more business-like including acquiring up-to-date computer systems and recruiting new doctors to join the practice—all of which was very expensive. Finally, as Peters noted, the Stark Law which Congress passed in 1992 changed the relationship between physicians and hospitals. This law regulates potential conflict of interest—the result of some physicians having investment in or compensatory relationship with a hospital. In other words, Stark made it hard for Avera McKennan to help an independent McGreevy Clinic. Thus, on January 1, 2006, McGreevy Clinic, with the support of 80 percent of the clinic's doctors, formally became part of Avera McKennan and, in 2009, was renamed Avera McGreevy Clinic. Ultimately, as a result of McGreevy Clinic joining Avera Health, the system expanded to have over 270 physicians throughout its network. Dave Flicek spoke of the McGreevy relationship: "They were good partners, good neighbors, good friends. And so it was a much easier relationship. And, again, they had a great culture, and we didn't want to change that culture. We wanted them to marry our culture, so that we could learn from one another."[226]

David Flicek was involved at the earliest stages of creating a regional medical system.[227] Flicek noted there were many reasons that both hospitals and physicians sought to unite in a larger health network. For some it was the increasingly complex technology while for others it was the changing nature of medicine. As a result of this approach, Avera McKennan has partnered with hospitals and clinics as far south as Chambers, Neb., and as far north as Ellendale, N.D. Flicek described the Avera philosophy behind inviting physicians, clinics or even hospitals into the larger system: "Our philosophy and really the Sisters' philosophy is that we meet people where they want to be met" and for Flicek this meant ensuring that "they need to know who we are" and are comfortable with the mission of the organization. "We don't see this as a takeover acquisition; we see it as a learning relationship going forward."[228]

To the present, Avera McKennan employs over **285 physicians** while offering privileges to over 500 and it partners with over **70 clinics** and **14 regional hospitals.**

Avera McKennan's network of hospitals, clinics and other service providers is in turn just one part of the Avera Health system, which includes nearly **300 health care entities** in **95 communities** throughout the **five-state** region.

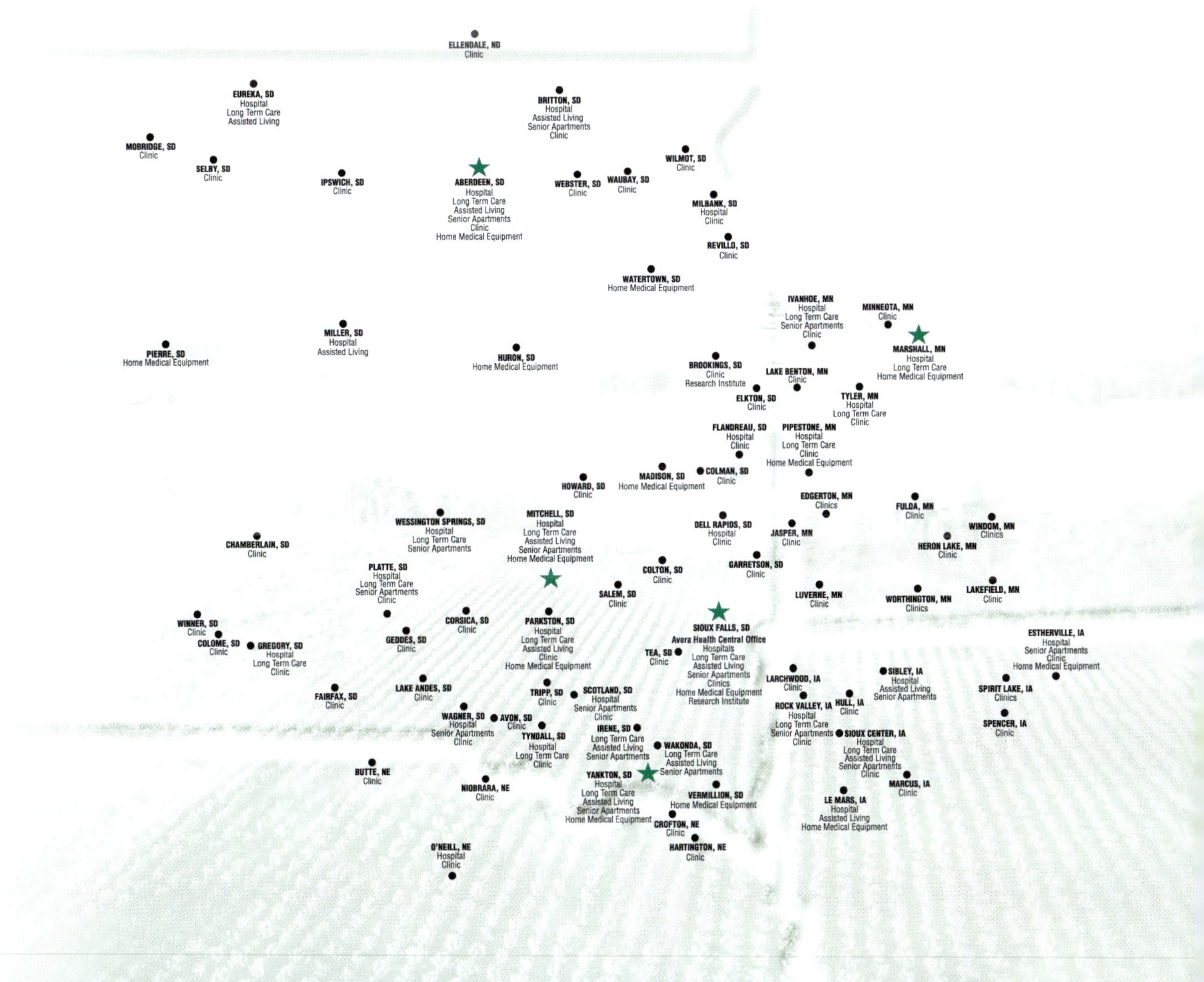

ELLENDALE, ND
Clinic

EUREKA, SD
Hospital
Long Term Care
Assisted Living

BRITTON, SD
Hospital
Assisted Living
Senior Apartments
Clinic

WILMOT, SD
Clinic

MOBRIDGE, SD
Clinic

SELBY, SD
Clinic

IPSWICH, SD
Clinic

ABERDEEN, SD
Hospital
Long Term Care
Assisted Living
Senior Apartments
Clinic
Home Medical Equipment

WEBSTER, SD
Clinic

WAUBAY, SD
Clinic

MILBANK, SD
Hospital
Clinic

REVILLO, SD
Clinic

WATERTOWN, SD
Home Medical Equipment

IVANHOE, MN
Hospital
Long Term Care
Senior Apartments
Clinic

MINNEOTA, MN
Clinic

MILLER, SD
Hospital
Assisted Living

PIERRE, SD
Home Medical Equipment

HURON, SD
Home Medical Equipment

BROOKINGS, SD
Clinic
Research Institute

LAKE BENTON, MN
Clinic

MARSHALL, MN
Hospital
Long Term Care
Home Medical Equipment

ELKTON, SD
Clinic

TYLER, MN
Hospital
Long Term Care
Clinic

FLANDREAU, SD
Hospital
Clinic

PIPESTONE, MN
Hospital
Long Term Care
Clinic
Home Medical Equipment

MADISON, SD
Home Medical Equipment

COLMAN, SD
Clinic

HOWARD, SD
Clinic

EDGERTON, MN
Clinics

FULDA, MN
Clinic

WESSINGTON SPRINGS, SD
Hospital
Long Term Care
Senior Apartments

MITCHELL, SD
Hospital
Long Term Care
Assisted Living
Senior Apartments
Home Medical Equipment

DELL RAPIDS, SD
Hospital
Clinic

JASPER, MN
Clinic

WINDOM, MN
Clinics

HERON LAKE, MN
Clinic

CHAMBERLAIN, SD
Clinic

PLATTE, SD
Hospital
Long Term Care
Senior Apartments
Clinic

COLTON, SD
Clinic

GARRETSON, SD
Clinic

LAKEFIELD, MN
Clinic

SALEM, SD
Clinic

LUVERNE, MN
Clinic

WORTHINGTON, MN
Clinics

WINNER, SD
Clinic

COLOME, SD
Clinic

GREGORY, SD
Hospital
Long Term Care
Clinic

CORSICA, SD
Clinic

GEDDES, SD
Clinic

PARKSTON, SD
Hospital
Long Term Care
Assisted Living
Clinic
Home Medical Equipment

TEA, SD
Clinic

SIOUX FALLS, SD
Avera Health Central Office
Hospitals
Long Term Care
Assisted Living
Senior Apartments
Clinics
Home Medical Equipment
Research Institute

ESTHERVILLE, IA
Hospital
Senior Apartments
Clinic
Home Medical Equipment

LARCHWOOD, IA
Clinic

SIBLEY, IA
Hospital
Assisted Living
Senior Apartments

SPIRIT LAKE, IA
Clinics

FAIRFAX, SD
Clinic

LAKE ANDES, SD
Clinic

TRIPP, SD
Clinic

SCOTLAND, SD
Hospital
Senior Apartments
Clinic

ROCK VALLEY, IA
Hospital
Long Term Care
Senior Apartments
Clinic

HULL, IA
Clinic

SPENCER, IA
Clinic

WAGNER, SD
Hospital
Senior Apartments
Clinic

AVON, SD
Clinic

TYNDALL, SD
Hospital
Long Term Care
Clinic

IRENE, SD
Long Term Care
Assisted Living
Senior Apartments

WAKONDA, SD
Long Term Care
Assisted Living
Senior Apartments

SIOUX CENTER, IA
Hospital
Long Term Care
Assisted Living
Senior Apartments
Clinic

MARCUS, IA
Clinic

BUTTE, NE
Clinic

NIOBRARA, NE
Clinic

YANKTON, SD
Hospital
Long Term Care
Assisted Living
Senior Apartments
Home Medical Equipment

VERMILLION, SD
Home Medical Equipment

CROFTON, NE
Clinic

LE MARS, IA
Hospital
Assisted Living
Home Medical Equipment

O'NEILL, NE
Hospital
Clinic

HARTINGTON, NE
Clinic

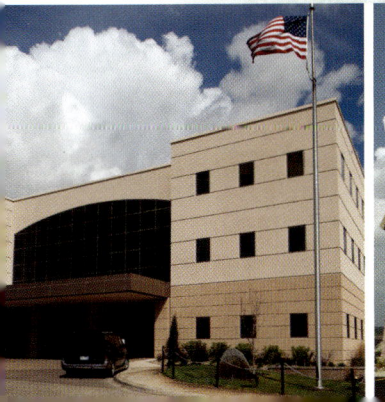
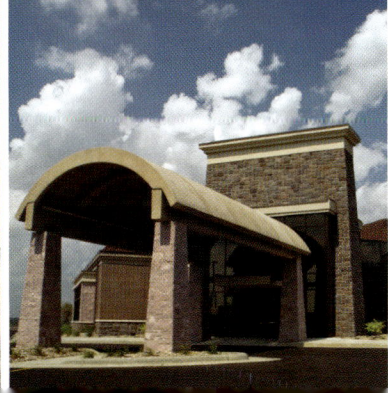
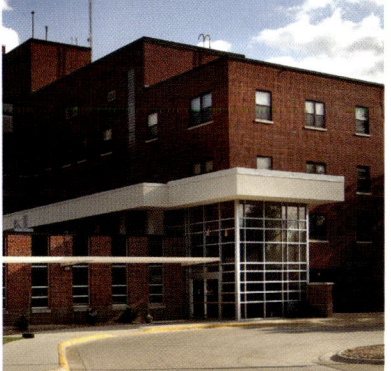
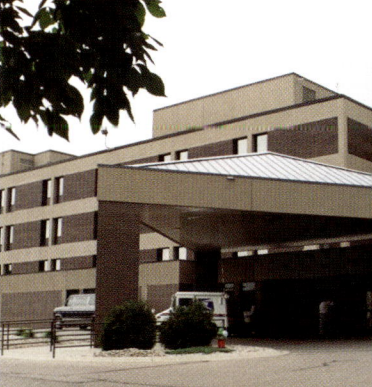

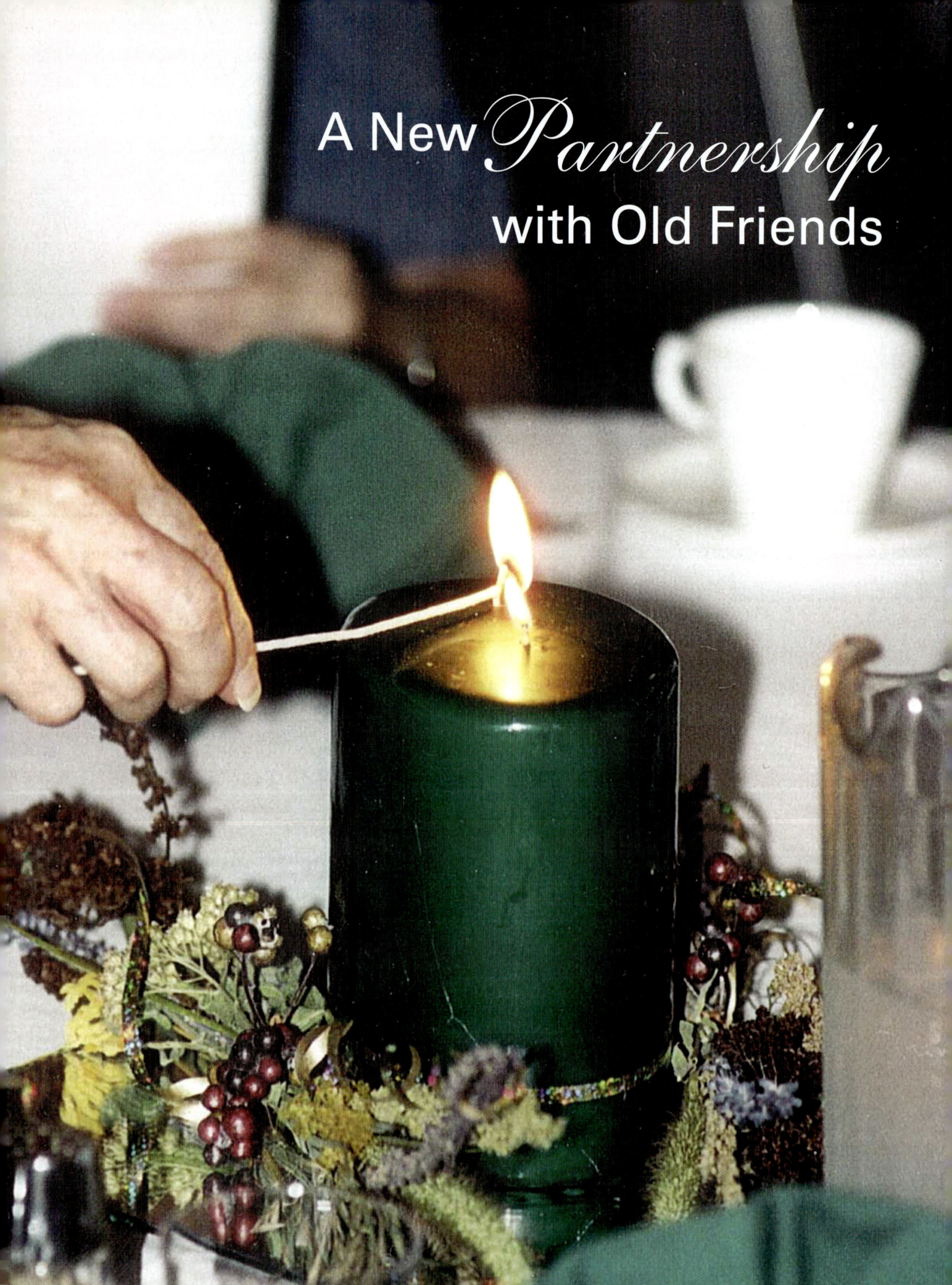

A New *Partnership*
with Old Friends

The Presentation Sisters of Aberdeen's Presentation Convent were neither the only order of Sisters that Bishop Martin Marty recruited to South Dakota—nor were they the only Sisters that Bishop Thomas O'Gorman asked to establish a hospital. The Benedictine Sisters, who were recruited to South Dakota by Marty in 1874, eventually settled in Yankton in 1889. In 1896 Bishop Thomas O'Gorman decided that the Yankton area needed a Catholic hospital and he asked the Benedictines of Yankton to staff one. Despite the fact that these women had been educators and had no Sisters who were trained nurses, they accepted O'Gorman's challenge—and within less than six months "the Hospital of the Sacred Heart—with 30 beds—was formally dedicated."[229]

Over the years as McKennan Hospital cared for the people of Sioux Falls while Sacred Heart Hospital cared for patients in Yankton, it became clear that there was room for collaboration. In 1978 the Presentation Sisters established Presentation Health Systems (PHS) "to combine the strengths of their individual institutions." Sister Colman Coakley became the first president of PHS' board of directors—which was made up of both religious and lay persons. This new organization sought to further share costs among Presentation hospitals including "legal affairs, personnel management, employee benefits administration, bill collection and risk management."[230] In 1987, the Benedictine Sisters formed the Benedictine Health System of Yankton. These two new organizations made it easier for both health systems to share ideas on health care management. The two increasingly had ties and by 1996 were sharing consulting, purchasing and other services.[231]

By the 1990s both the Presentation and Benedictine orders began to see that greater collaboration was an important part of each organization's survival. This developed as the Catholic Health Association of the United States called for greater cooperation among Catholic hospitals, nursing homes and clinics.[232] Nevertheless, as many realized, developing much closer ties between the two systems would

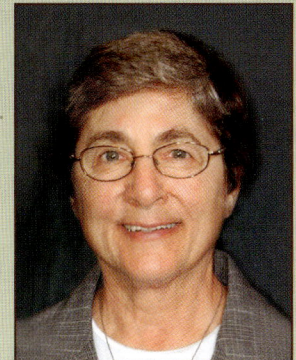

Sister Lynn Marie Welbig

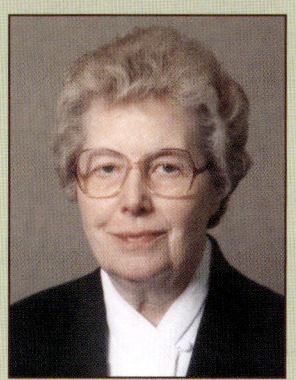

Sister Mary Denis Collins

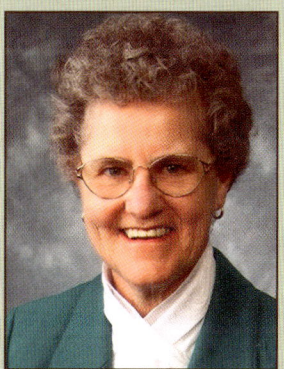

Sister Kate Crowley

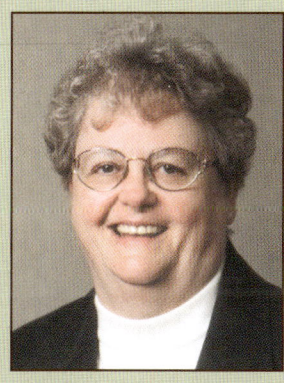

Sister Mildred Busch

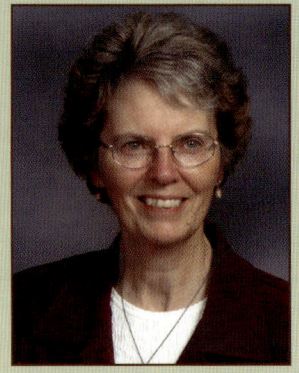

Sister Joyce Meyer

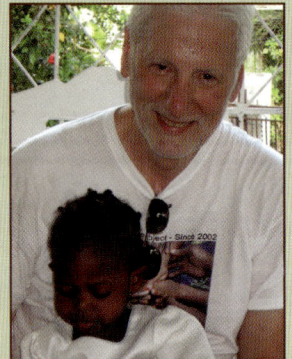

Bob Voglewede

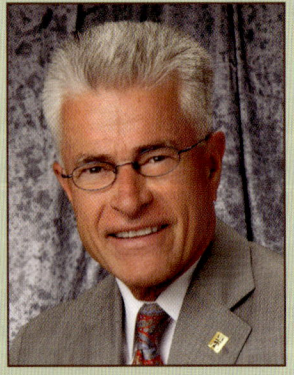

John Porter

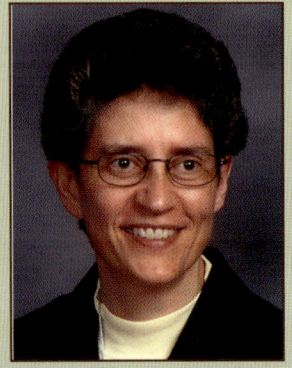

Sister Mary Thomas

be complicated. John Porter, president and CEO of Presentation Health Systems (eventually Avera Health) described it as a "lengthy intellectual and emotional process."[233] Serious and thoughtful discussion of how these two religious orders would join forces to strengthen their health care institutions began in 1996. In 2001 some of the sisters involved in the deliberations reflected upon the process. Sister Kate Crowley noted that the Benedictines "came to realize that we needed to go beyond our independence" and seek collaboration. Sister Lynn Marie Welbig of the Presentation Order stated that "it was a real discernment."

The challenge was that while both orders are, of course, Roman Catholic, they have very different cultures with very different histories. The Presentation Order was founded by an 18th century Irish woman who wanted those who joined her to be in the world working for the poor; the Benedictines, a much more contemplative order, trace their roots back to Benedict, a fifth century Italian monastic whose rule includes a commitment to stability, hospitality and prayer. Thus, reflected Sister Kate Crowley, the women needed to learn about each other's cultures before trying to unite their businesses.

In order to facilitate the change, the orders established a leadership council made up of 17 Sisters—12 Benedictines and five Presentations, who were to meet regularly. From this group, however, four women—two from each order, were selected to form a planning task force. In the summer of 2001 Bob Voglewede, Avera Health vice president for Mission Services, interviewed these women. Sisters Mary Denis Collins and Lynn Marie Welbig represented the Presentation Order while Sisters Mildred Busch and Kate Crowley represented the Benedictine Order.[234] Sister Lynn Marie noted that as the women got to know each other, they recognized that this was more than establishing a mere partnership: "We created a new entity. It is like a union…a marriage. It is a new thing with a new personality. Now Avera Health is going to go forward with a monastic and an apostolic identity. I think that is just a very rich concept."

Nevertheless, joining forces was a challenge for both communities. There were expressions of concern. Sister Mary Denis Collins recalled that there were questions from both congregations as to why they should make such a change. "What will it look like? Are we moving out of health care?" However, Sister Mary Denis also noted that such questions diminished as the two congregations came to know each other better. Sister Kate Crowley reflected on the process and felt that, for the Benedictine Sisters, what made the experience a positive one was when the Presentation Sisters spoke of what co-sponsorship meant to them: "They said they wanted us to be partners and not to worry about who brought what to the table. That, I must say, just overwhelmed us. And once that understanding began to take hold, the rest followed."

had changed; she stated that the name change "reflects the mission of helping people stay healthy rather than just taking care of them when they're ill."[236] In 2009 Sister Mary Thomas, Avera McKennan senior vice president for Mission Services, reflected on the creation of Avera Health and stated that there was a grieving process for all of the Sisters but, in the end, "they realized this was always the ministry of Jesus and they needed to do this because it was the next call...this was the next stage of this ministry. And they responded as they had with all the other stages before: generously."[237]

The careful consideration that went into the change did not go unnoticed by employees. David Flicek, chief administrative officer of Avera Medical Group, reflected on the work by the two religious communities:

After two years of discussion and discernment, the Presentation Sisters of Aberdeen and the Benedictine Sisters of Yankton entered into an agreement to co-sponsor Avera Health.

"The name is derived from the Latin word, "avere," which means "to be well."[235]

The challenges, including a sense of loss, were still at the surface when the name change was featured in the *Argus Leader* on March 12, 1998. "'We have mixed feelings,' noted Sister Joyce Meyer, president of the Sisters of the Presentation of the Blessed Virgin Mary, about the Presentation name disappearing from the health system." Nevertheless, Sister Joyce went on to state that the new name was "inclusive of all our partners that are part of [the] system." In addition, Sister Joyce noted how much the world of medicine

"They wanted to really make sure that their beliefs were the same, that they could work together...and honestly, I think the credit is to the Sisters. If it wasn't for the Sisters' forethought, I don't think it would have been as successful."[238] In 2008, nurse Becky Severson who has worked for Avera McKennan since 1979 spoke on the change to the Avera name. Hesitant at first, she said she soon saw it as a good thing and, "I think it really has helped create a sense of unity."[239]

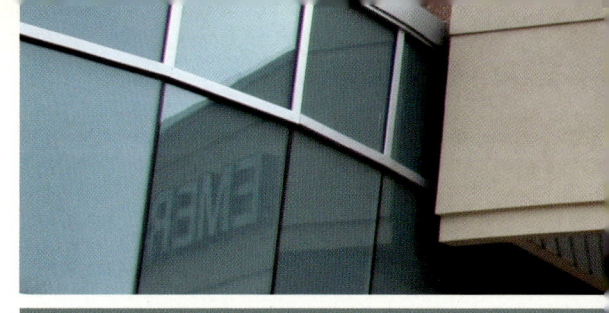

In 2004, Avera McKennan announced that it would spend $8 million to reconstruct its aging emergency room.

Treating Patients in a
HIGH-TECH WORLD

The new design sought to create a place that would feel less like an emergency room and more a welcoming environment for patients and their families. As part of the renovation, the ambulance area was expanded and the Emergency Department (ED) enlarged to three times its previous size. The renovation added more patient rooms, resulting in a total of 16; all of them private. In order to make the architectural design more efficient, Avera McKennan studied a number of emergency rooms around the country. A team of full-time emergency physicians who are all residency trained and board-certified in emergency medicine provide patient care and make Avera McKennan the only hospital in the state and region to offer such experienced personnel.[240]

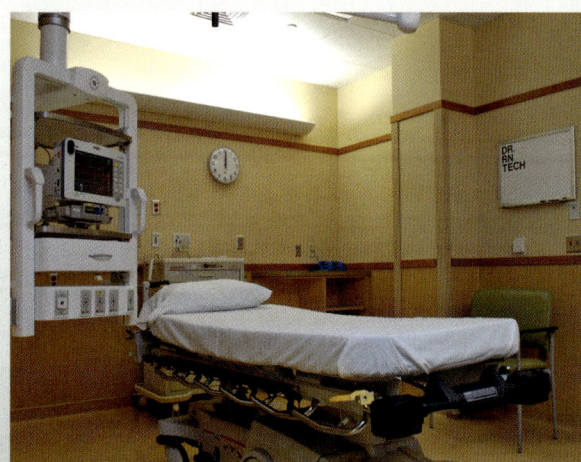

The Emergency Department was one of the first departments to which Avera McKennan applied the LEAN process.[241] An innovative architectural design to enhance efficiency and improve patient flow ultimately saved the hospital $1.25 million in construction costs.[242] In an even more significant innovation, the Emergency Department now uses technology to improve patient care both in Sioux Falls and in emergency rooms around the state. Avera Health launched *e*Emergency in October of 2009. It links Avera McKennan's ED with other hospitals across the state, allowing Avera to serve as one of the first health care sites in the country to offer rural hospitals 24-hour emergency services across a broadband network.

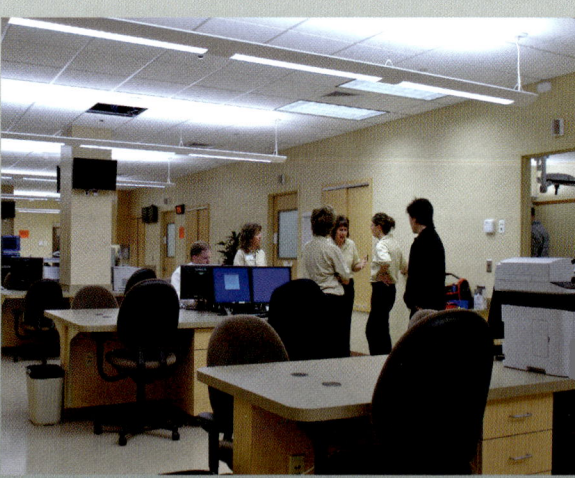

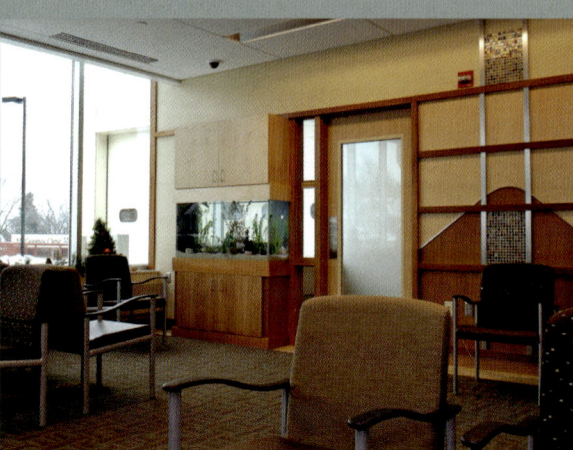

Staffed by a team of emergency-trained specialists, the 24-hour service allows facilities to have both support and consultation services. With the push of a button, staff at a rural facility initiate a two-way video conference with emergency personnel in Sioux Falls.[243] Beginning with eight rural sites, Avera continues to add hospitals to the list.[244]

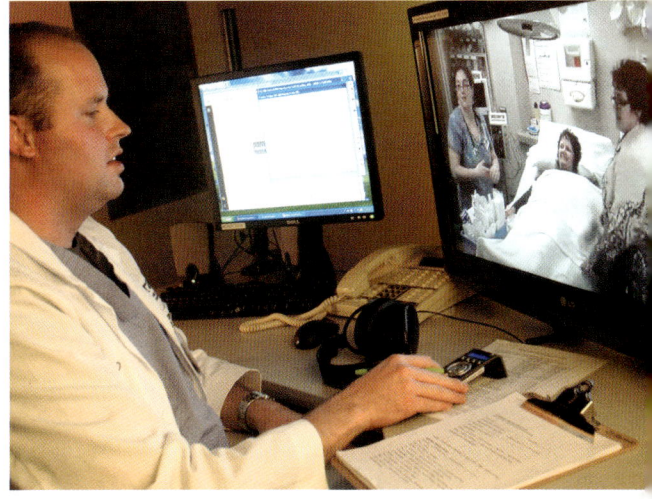

This use of technology for long-distance care, which is broadly called telemedicine, evolved during the latter half of the 20th century. The first successful use of video communications was documented by the University of Nebraska in 1959. Over the next four decades, the process slowly evolved. NASA played a leading role in telemedicine and along with the U.S. Indian Health Service and the Lockheed Missile and Space Company, initiated telemedicine to provide medical services to astronauts and residents of an isolated Native American reservation. While the process was hampered by high transmission costs in the 1980s, as these decreased over the next decade the use of telemedicine spread. There are many benefits to telemedicine including an estimated reduction in medical care costs of $36 billion annually. In addition to improving access to specialists and enhancing decision-making for all parties, telemedicine empowers patients enabling them to make more "informed decisions regarding their health care." Significantly, if patients are able to remain at their local hospitals, they often have a better response to treatment as a result of having family and friends close by and able to visit regularly.[245]

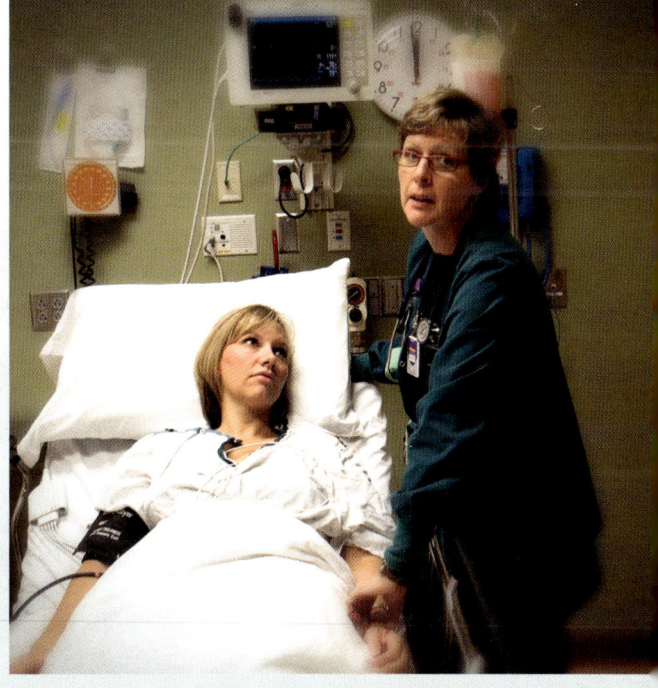

Avera McKennan's use of telemedicine is much broader than emergency care and its involvement with telemedicine dates back to the early 1990s when it recognized that such technology

Avera Health launched
eEmergency
in October of 2009

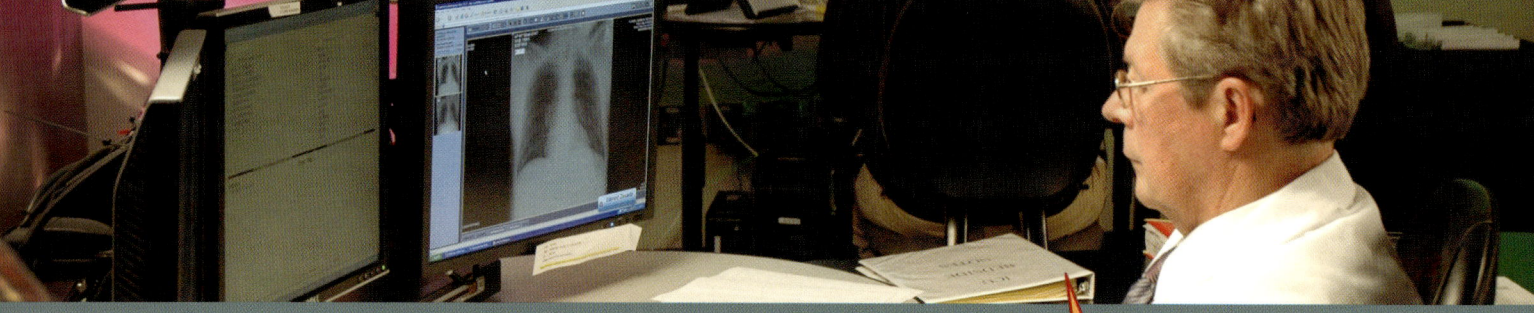

Dr. Edward Zawada

Health Care's MOST WIRED.® Winner 2009

would enable it to better support the rural community. Avera Health's telehealth services have expanded to what is today known as Avera eCARE, a suite of innovative technology applications leveraged by highly trained staff to extend 24-hour access in rural areas to specialty care physicians and pharmacists. Other applications include eICU, eStroke, ePharmacy, ePrescribing, Avera HealtheCARE electronic medical record, and eConsult–interactive consultations offered at more than 50 locations by over 30 providers in 14 different medical specialty areas. Avera eCARE has received many grants over the years including, in 2009, a $6 million grant from the Leona M. and Harry B. Helmsley Charitable Trust.[246]

All of Avera's predictions of what telemedicine would bring to rural doctors and patients, including better care and decreased cost, have now come true.[247] An example is Avera eICU® CARE, which connects specially trained personnel in critical care with health facilities in order to offer additional support and monitoring of patients who are in an ICU bed in a rural locale. Nationwide studies also show that telehealth care reduces mortality and shortens hospital stays.[248] Through eICU, implemented in 2004, there has been a nearly 40 percent reduction in the need to transfer patients from their local hospital. There has also been a reduction in the length of stay in small community hospitals ICUs and local physicians suggest that they feel that they can provide better care as a

result of having access to Avera eICU® CARE. All of this, in the long run, improves care and reduces cost. Dr. Edward Zawada, medical director of Avera eICU® CARE, noted: "The health care quality and safety benefits of ICU telemedicine have been well-documented. What is becoming evident are the significant financial benefits that can accrue from this improved quality. Equally important are benefits like less stress on rural physicians and nurses, and higher patient and family satisfaction."[249]

In 2010, for the 12th year in a row, *Hospitals & Health Networks* magazine named Avera among the "Most Wired." For the seventh year in a row the magazine named Avera among the "Most Wireless." Since the inception of these awards, Avera is the only health system in the nation to make both lists every year. Avera McKennan has become a regional leader in telemedicine. This was exemplified by the fact that the American Telemedicine Association awarded Avera's telehealth program the Presidential Institutional Award in 2009. This award came only five years after Avera McKennan established "the first eICU in a Midwestern rural setting to provide this life-saving service to Critical Access Hospitals."[250]

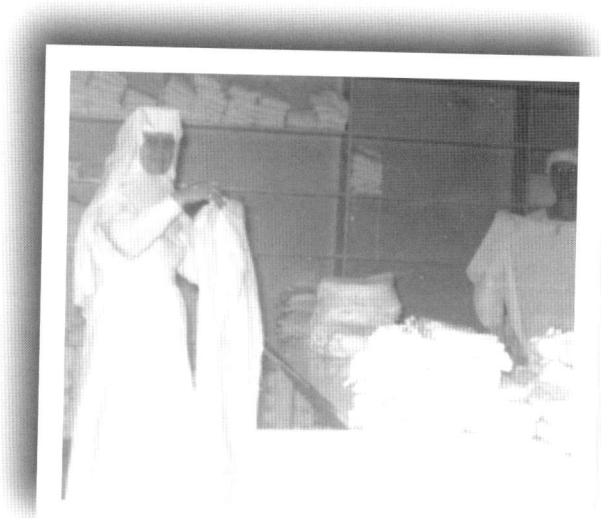

Sister David Dorn

A Thing of Beauty...

Of the many departments in the hospital, there are some that steadily work behind the scenes and, while sometimes overlooked, are no less important. When McKennan Hospital opened in 1911, it had an on-site laundry connected to the hospital via an underground tunnel. The laundry was under the leadership of Irish immigrant Sister Philomena Brennan who ensured that fresh linens were delivered daily to the floors. According to records, between 1911 and 1932, the laundry had a three-roll mangle, two-hand operated presses, one wooden washer and two extractors. The hospital's first dryer was installed in 1932.

In 1940, Sister David Dorn took charge of the laundry. A native of Adrian, Minn., Miss Martha Dorn entered the Presentation Order in 1932. When Sister Dorn arrived, McKennan was still using some of the machinery from 1916—though in 1951 the hospital added another washer because the laundry's 10 employees were now working seven days a week.

It is clear is that Sister David ran a tight ship in the laundry. Dr. Richard Hosen, a pediatrician originally with Donohoe Clinic, immediately noticed the laundry's good work: "When you were in the hospital you were in the Sisters' home, and it showed. In the surgery suite and the OB dressing rooms, the scrubs were all neatly folded and sized." Ms. Madonna Clark, who worked in Medical Records at McKennan Hospital from 1944 to 1984, spoke fondly of Sister David and remembered that: "her laundry was a thing of beauty."

In January of 1972, Sister David's "thing of beauty" was retired as the hospital closed the laundry, setting aside the steam operated presses and stainless steel washers and dryers. The machinery was well aged and the space was needed for a new addition. The hospital's linens were now sent to a commercial laundry. In 1982, after 45 years of service, Sister David retired from working at McKennan Hospital and she passed away in 1994.

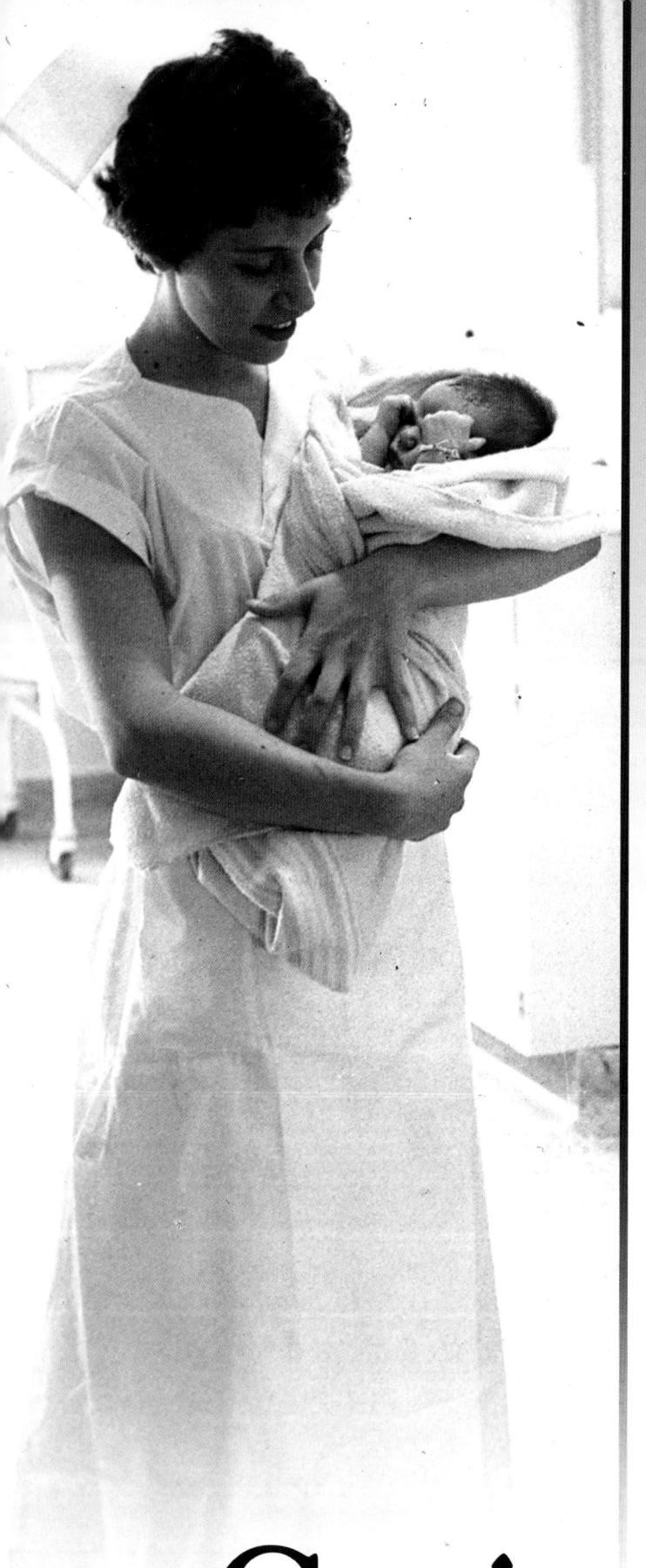

In 1954, the *Argus Leader* featured an article about a McKennan nurse who had clearly made a difference for mothers and their babies. Sister Mary Matthew Brady was an obstetric supervisor at McKennan Hospital between 1932 and 1946 who brought much comfort to those for whom she cared. Born Rose Mary Brady in County Cavan, Ireland, in 1903, she graduated from St. Luke's School of Nursing in 1927. The article reflected on Sister Matthew's life before she developed brain cancer and died in 1954 at the age of 51. Many sought to honor her life and recognize her work. The *Argus Leader* reported that patients, doctors and nurses alike were devoted to Sister Matthew for her skill and kindness.[251] Although Dr. Russell Orr could not recall the Sister's name, maybe it was Sister Matthew who helped Orr, a long-time Sioux Falls obstetrician, when he was just starting to practice. As Orr recalled:

> The average young family practitioner was released to the public with little experience…and she was so intelligent and so experienced that when you'd come over to the hospital and a patient had a problem, she would say to you, 'Doctor, I know you knew that if this lady was having some breathing problem, you would have a couple of units of blood available and an IV running, so I've arranged all that for you.' And it would be done. And if somebody showed signs of toxemia pregnancy, she'd immediately have the equipment in place and going by the time you'd get over to the hospital. She'd say, 'I know this is your routine.' So she was continually educating all of us.[252]

Caring for Life

Another physician, Dr. W. F. Sercl stated of Sister Matthew, "I know of no person who has given so much of themselves to the people of Sioux Falls as Sister Matthew. The most she ever asked for was an occasional Hail Mary in return." Clearly Sister Matthew had great compassion, and, as the *Argus Leader* noted, "many an unwed mother owes her ability to cope with the world to Sister Matthew, whose cult of worshippers is limited to no one religion."[253]

Yet, it was for the infants that Sister Matthew had a particular dedication and she gave equal attention to each. Eleanor "Mickey" Billion, a 1942 graduate of McKennan's School of Nursing, knew Sister Matthew and recalled that she would beg post-partum mothers for breast milk. "If there were children in the nursery that weren't doing well...she'd go around and beg for breast milk...and use it for the babies that needed it."[254] After her untimely death, there was such an outpouring from her many thankful friends that McKennan Hospital established the Sister Matthew Fund. Proceeds, that reached nearly $2,100, went toward the purchase of delivery tables and equipment for four nurseries in the hospital's new wing.[255]

In 1961, upon McKennan Hospital's 50th anniversary, the *Argus Leader* discussed how McKennan's maternity ward and its 40 bassinets allowed the hospital to offer each child individual care. This was a far cry from the hospital's earliest days when, as recalled by one McKennan nurse, "infants were delivered in their mother's room and...the nursery for newborns or sick babies was wherever a room was available."[256] At this time, mothers and babies stayed in the hospital for about two weeks. Nurse Albena Reinke, who first began in McKennan's nursery in 1956, recalled that she and an aid put five babies into a cart of stainless steel containers and wheeled them out to mothers.[257]

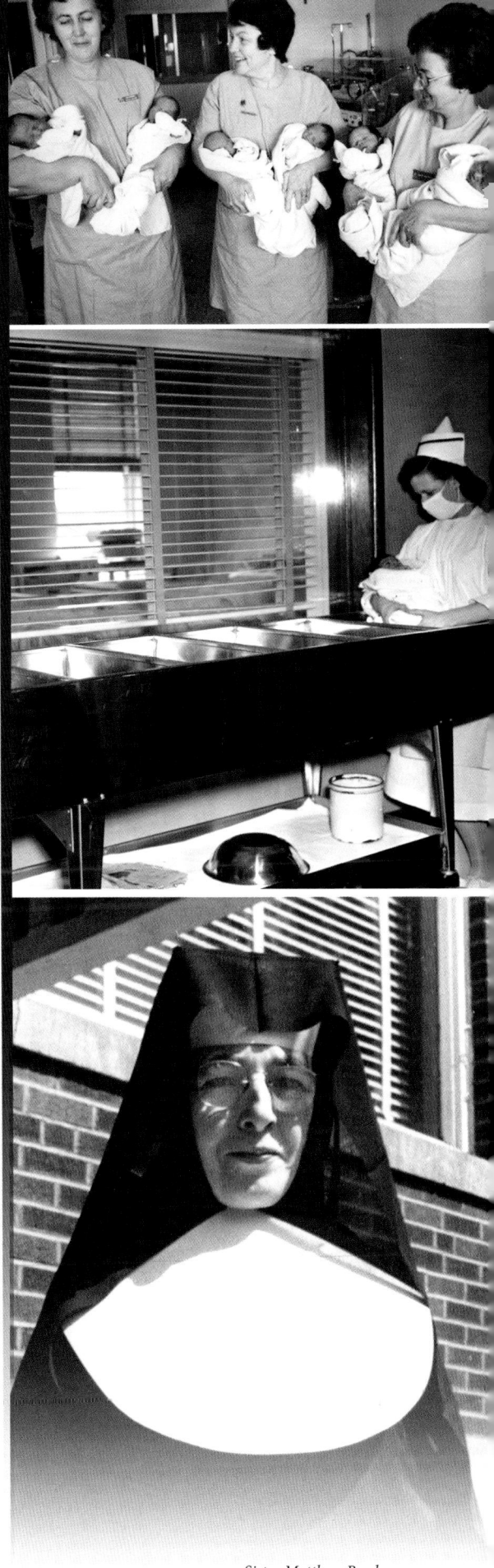

Sister Matthew Brady

In the early 1970s, in order to ease the transition for new mothers, McKennan Hospital collaborated with the nursing department at Augustana College to have junior-year nursing students gain clinical experience by emphasizing care of newborns and their mothers. Students spent time in labor and delivery rooms, the nursery and with mothers. Each student nurse was assigned to a specific patient beginning an "association with a maternity patient during the latter's prenatal visits at the physician's office." For new mothers this program was meant to bring further comfort, while for experienced mothers the hospital's hope was that they could offer insights to the nursing students. At about this time the hospital also built special labor and post-birth rooms in which nurses monitored babies during their first hours of life.[258]

In 1989, McKennan ushered in a new era of delivery by offering the LDRP room (labor, delivery, recovery and postpartum) which allowed a woman to stay in the same room in which she delivered the baby. While McKennan began with two, it planned to convert all of its rooms. Fathers were now in the delivery rooms— a change from earlier in the century when men waited outside to hear the news of baby's birth but the hospital still maintained a retreat called the "Daddy's Den," where anxious fathers might seek comradeship. Becky Severson, who began at McKennan as an OB nurse in 1979, recalled going to the "Den" to find a father who had already been informed that he had a daughter. "He had gone out to the Daddy's Den to call family and by the time he left the delivery room the doctor said, 'I think there's another one coming.' So I run out to find him and he was on the phone saying, 'We've had a baby girl.' And I said, 'You have two girls!' He had this stunned look on his face. I still remember that 'deer in the headlight' look." Severson, program manager for Avera McKennan Women's and Children's, recalls her more than 30 years at McKennan fondly, and as a new nurse she never expected to spend her career in obstetrics:

> When I first started, I asked a nurse how long she had been here and she said 15 years. My first thought was, "Wow! Are you old." My second thought was, "Boy are you in a rut!" And here I am almost 30 years later, having worked in one capacity or another in OB. I think that particularly in an area like OB, it's such an honor! You get to help bring new souls into the world. It never gets old. You're here at a very special time in parents' lives. It isn't always a happy occasion, but even then, hopefully you're there and can still make it as good as possible for them.[259]

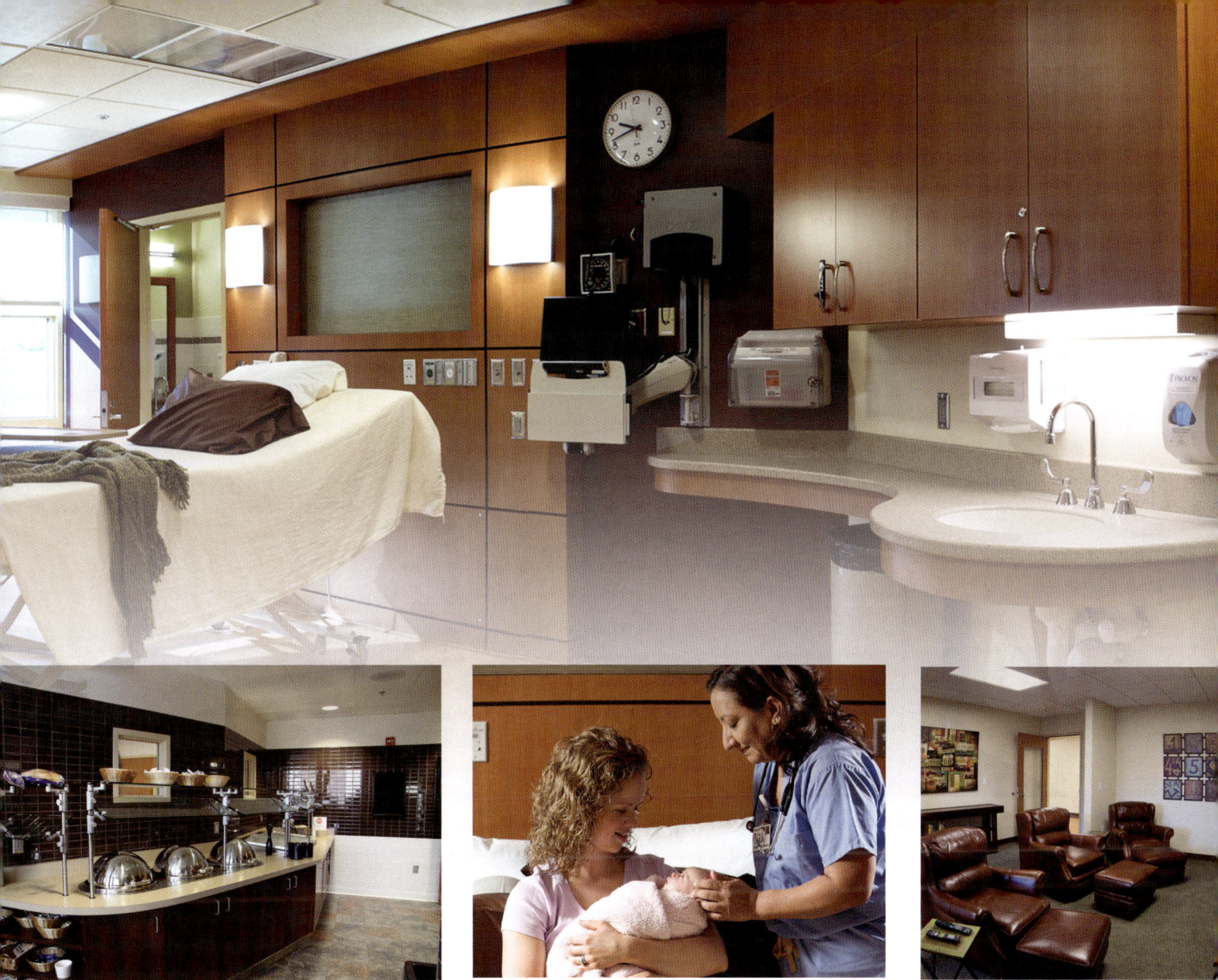

To further advance the care of mothers and babies, in 1992 McKennan announced that the hospital had decided to build a two-story addition to double the space for maternity services. McKennan had experienced impressive growth in labor and delivery; between 1987 and 1991, deliveries increased 21 percent and these numbers continued to rise. It became clear that the hospital needed to modernize its facilities, especially given that some of the services were still housed in a section of the 1919 structure. Thus, as part of the hospital's earlier commitment, it also announced that it now planned to build some 15 to 20 LDRPs.[260]

The hospital continued to adapt to changing technology as well as maintain its long history in women's and pediatric care. As the population of Sioux Falls continued to grow, it recognized that it needed to further expand its maternal facilities. On September 4, 2008, Avera McKennan opened a post-partum addition to its Women's Center. Still hosting a "Dad's Den," the Women's Center focuses on the care and comfort of mother and child, and thus not only does the center have the latest technology, it also includes an on-site café and post-partum spa services. In 2009, births at Avera McKennan increased by 13 percent.[261]

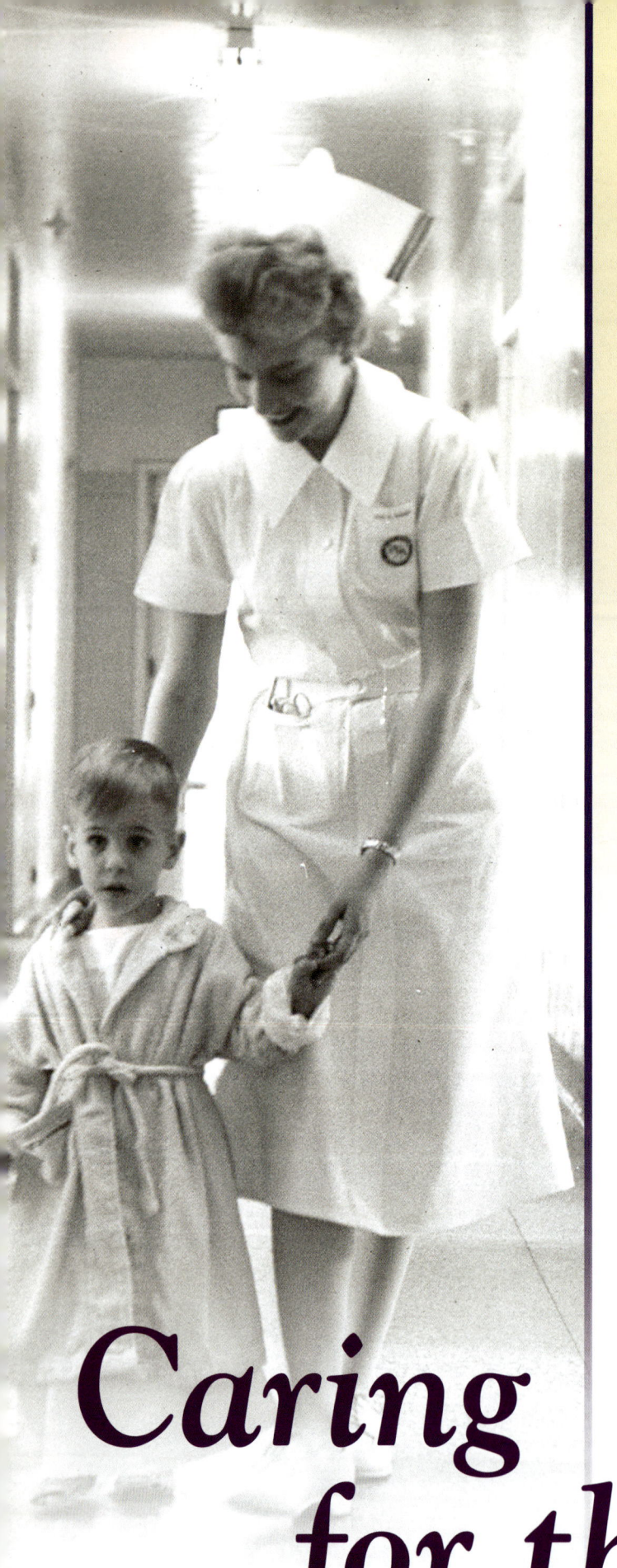

Helen McKennan, herself a pioneer, would have been proud to see McKennan Hospital take the road less traveled with regard to the types of medical care the hospital offered. In 1958, when few in the state were offering such services, McKennan devoted its fourth floor to patients needing psychiatric care. The only psychiatric facility in the area under hospital management, McKennan dedicated 27 beds on the fourth floor and built a "well-equipped kitchen, supervisor's office, service education office, psychiatrist's office, consultation room, treatment room, nurse's station, combined day room and dining room." The *Argus Leader* lamented that while patients would no longer have to travel elsewhere for assistance, the number of beds the ward contained would probably be far below the demand. Nevertheless, the paper cheered the fact that an occupational therapy department would be included on the wing offering "woodworking, ceramics, weaving, art work and other activities vital to rehabilitation."[262]

In 1976 an *Argus Leader* article discussed the psychiatric services McKennan offered noting that it was seeking to change the emphasis to mental health as opposed to mental illness. The hope was to reduce patient time in the hospital through having mental health workers offer nonjudgmental counseling services in "a pleasant atmosphere" which was comfortably furnished and staffed by persons "in non-uniform street dress who are easily accessible to talk with, play games and participate in all forms of therapy with the patients."

Caring for the Spirit

Char Herman, at that time a clinical nurse specialist for McKennan's Mental Health Department, said that: "We work toward helping the individual help himself, and direct therapy toward increasing self-confidence and sense of self-worth."[263]

McKennan continued to expand its psychiatric care. In 1978, McKennan Hospital and the Department of Psychiatry at the University of South Dakota School of Medicine jointly administered an adolescent psychiatric care program that sought to maintain family involvement with 13-to 18-year-old patients and provide a safe setting that also offered recreational opportunities.[264] In 2006, culminating Avera McKennan's nearly 50 years in mental health services, the hospital opened a $32 million 110-bed facility that serves the needs of persons of all ages.[265] Now the largest in the region, the Avera Behavioral Health Center is on par with Fairview Mental Health Services and the Mayo Clinic, both of Minnesota.[266]

As the Avera Behavioral Health Center opened, Steve Lindquist, assistant vice president for Avera McKennan Behavioral Health Services, noted: "Our facility has become known nationally as a setting for the leading edge for psychiatric treatment facilities." Offering inpatient and outpatient care, the medical director, Dr. Matthew Stanley, a psychiatrist with Avera University Psychiatry Associates and Avera Behavioral Health Services, stated: "Avera's commitment to behavioral health stems from our belief in being compassionate caregivers." Seeking to further de-stigmatize mental illness, the Avera Behavioral Health Center sought to integrate unique art and architecture into a facility that encourages the healing of mind, body and spirit.[267]

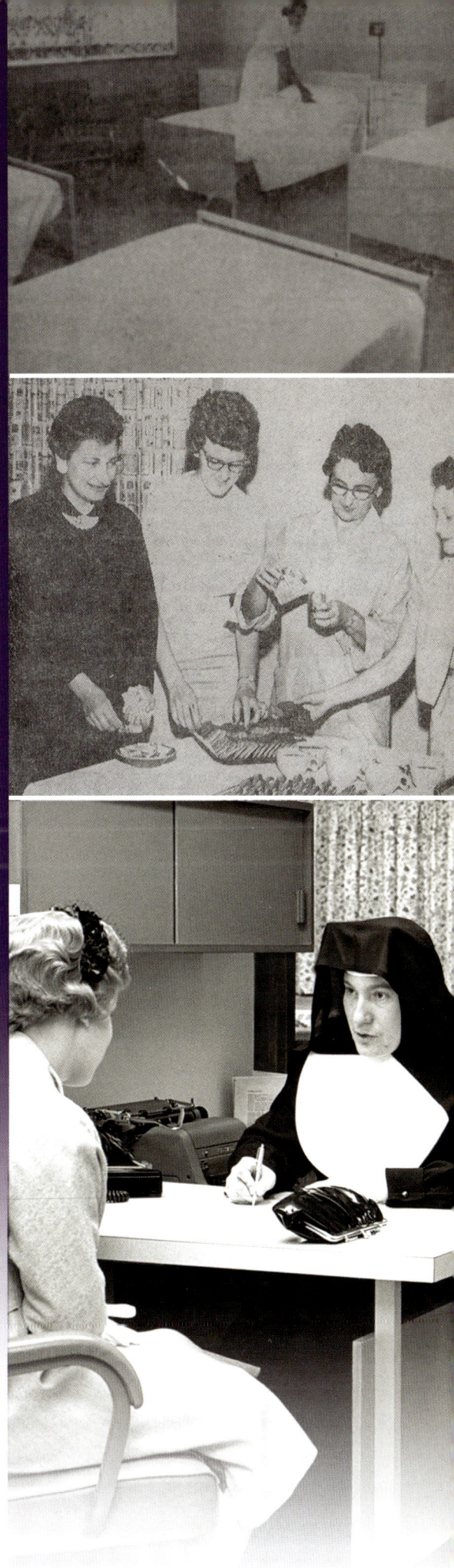

The art in the building was not an afterthought but an integral part of the design. As Fred Slunecka stated, the art was planned at the same time as the building itself: "We gave the artists the color palette and the rough architectural designs." The theme was based on the Bible verse "Rise on the Wings of Dawn" and this can be intuited from Terri Schuver's 15-foot steel sculpture that sits at the front entrance and is titled "Butterfly Breeze." Said Schuver: "I wanted it to be comforting and positive, uplifting and non-threatening, because that's how we would want people to feel as they enter or leave the building." The Avera Behavioral Health Center offers care to persons in all stages; catering to the needs of growing children while offering help to adults.[268]

Citing the Avera Behavioral Health Center and its work in mental health care, the American Hospital Association and McKesson announced in July of 2008 that Avera McKennan was one of only four hospitals in the country recognized through the Quest for Quality Prize Program with a "citation of merit" for "leadership and innovation in quality, safety and commitment in patient care." Avera McKennan received this award after several days of inspection regarding both how the hospital does its work but also "how we interact with our community."[269]

As the Avera Behavioral Health Center continues its work, it has become home to the state's only genetic lab, the Avera Institute for Human Behavioral Genetics (IHBG). A key goal is to "combine genetic and environmental principles with an aim toward health and wellness in children, families and communities." Helping to launch this project was internationally-known child psychiatrist and genetic researcher Dr. James Hudziak. Hudziak stated: "While the presence of a certain gene can increase the chances of developing an illness, it doesn't guarantee that outcome...some type of environmental factor must also be present to act as a trigger."[270] The environment around the child can be negative, such as abuse, or positive such as good nutrition and participation in athletic or artistic activities. How nature and nurture interact is the question.

The program was imagined by Drs. Matthew Stanley and Timothy Soundy. They approached Fred Slunecka who found it "an exciting prospect. Together we can build a stronger framework for social health. Together we can design a better prevention and treatment approach for children and families with psychiatric disorders." In 2008, Avera McKennan supplied $1.5 million to the project with the hopes of raising additional money through private donations. The IHBG project is collaborative and includes partnerships with the South Dakota State University College of Pharmacy, the University of South Dakota, the University of South Dakota Sanford School of Medicine Department of Psychiatry and other local community organizations.[271]

While the scientific track is conducted by Avera Institute for Human Behavioral Genetics (IHBG), the "environmental" track is administered by the Avera Family Wellness Program that works with preschool children in order to keep them well and healthy.[272] Among other things, the children were taught violin, offered art classes and tai chi in an effort, says Ryan Hansen, clinical research director

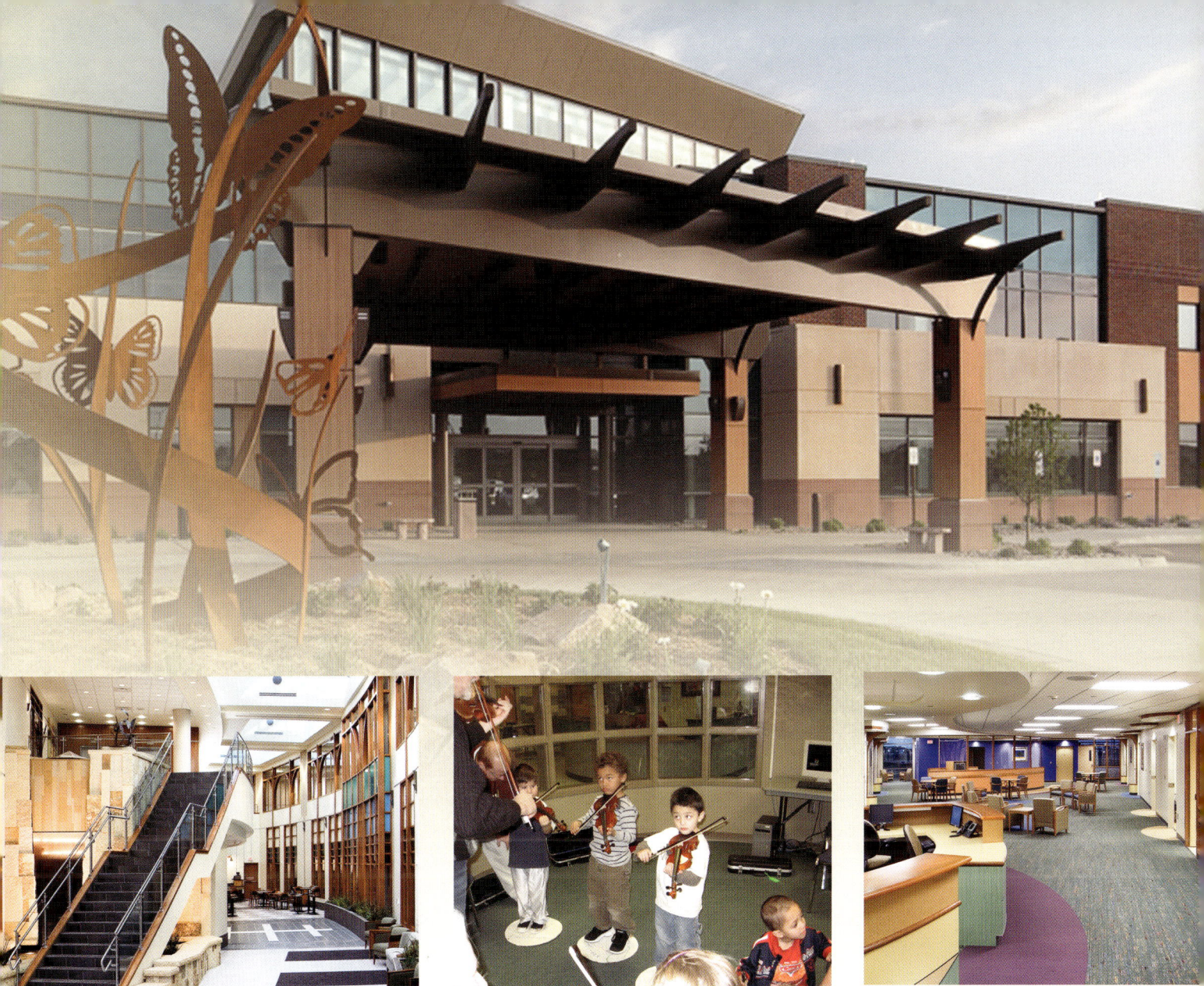

for the Avera Research Institute, to "influence behavior in positive ways within young children that will allow them to be more successful early in life." It is hoped that such directed activities will reduce the stress these youngsters experience and, as a result, encouragebetter behavior.

The program's first year was a great success and culminated in a March recital held at Sioux Falls Washington Pavilion where the children performed alongside the South Dakota Symphony Youth Orchestra.[273] In its second year, the program moved to Hawarden Elementary School and limited its focus to violin training, "from which the first-year data was the most encouraging. Children enrolled in the program demonstrated a decrease in negative behaviors." Finally, in addition to providing preschool children with the skills to have a positive educational future, the Avera Family Wellness Program provides the parents with a "personal health coach" who works with them in making good choices for the welfare of their children and, if need be, the children and families are offered counseling.[274]

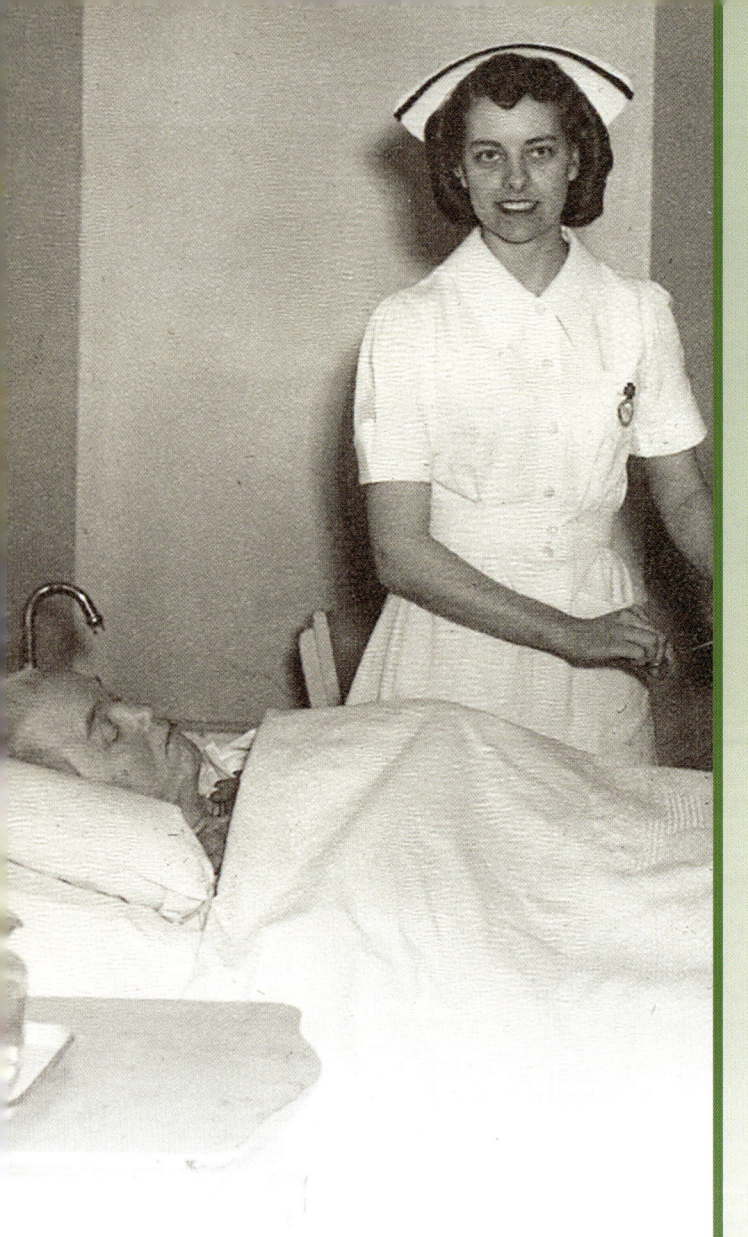

In 1906, Helen McKennan spent her last days of life in her home surrounded by her friends and family. McKennan, according to Dr. Perkins, knew she was dying and prepared herself for this eventuality by laying out the plans for a park and hospital in her will. We do not know who cared for Helen McKennan in her last days, but her will left money to her former "attendants and employees," some of whom probably sought to ease her suffering.[275]

Helen McKennan had the good fortune to die in her own home but it was only in the latter half of the 20th century that there developed increased recognition of the humanity, wisdom and dignity of providing a comfortable, non-institutional environment in which persons can spend their last days. While the history of hospice care goes back, at minimum, to the fifth century, during the 19th and 20th centuries there can be found increasing examples of charitable establishments that cared for the dying. In the late 1960s, Dr. Cicely Saunders, who helped to found St. Christopher's Hospice in London, brought her program to the United States where it quickly caught on. By the early 1970s, the first stages of this modern hospice movement began in earnest in the United States with care being provided

Caring for the Community:
Hospice & Home Care

primarily in the home. In 1982, as part of amendments to the Social Security Act, the Hospice Medicare Benefit was established and became permanent in 1985. In 1995, the American Board of Hospice and Palliative Medicine was created and offered examinations for physicians to become certified in this specialty. All along the way, hospice care continued to grow. In 2005, more than 1.2 million people received hospice care in the U.S. alone. In addition, "from 1985 to 2005, the number of hospice sites increased from approximately 1,500 to more than 4,000," while between 2000 and 2006, the number of palliative care programs saw a 96 percent increase.[276]

In 1982, McKennan Hospital created a plan to support terminally ill patients and allow them to die in the comfort of their own home. In addition to family members, friends and health care providers, the hospital supplied "a trained volunteer…to each hospice family, spending at least four hours a week helping out." The volunteer did "light housework, played cards, read aloud or other needed duties." After the patient's death, the volunteer kept in touch with the family for the following year. In the mid 1980s, McKennan's hospice care expanded and the hospital first opened a four bed in-house hospice unit. In addition to respite for the families, in-hospital hospice offered, "great physical, emotional and spiritual support, opportunities for pain management and care for the side effects of treatment (and the dying process)." Decorated to offer a home-like experience, this in-hospital hospice was the first of its kind in South Dakota and offered an "interdisciplinary" approach which involved nurses, therapists, social workers, volunteers, the

patient's family and doctors. Volunteers received more extensive training and assisted with a variety of tasks that helped the patient as well as the family.[277]

While today Avera McKennan continues to offer inpatient and in-home hospice care, in 2006 Avera McKennan announced that it would build a $3.6 million hospice center on the grounds of the Avera Prince of Peace Retirement Community. The Sioux Falls Catholic Diocese opened Prince of Peace in 1986 and the Presentation Order managed it until 1994, when it merged with McKennan Hospital.[278] The retirement community expanded over the years and offers assisted and independent living in addition to long-term care. Michael and Kathy Dougherty announced that they would donate $1 million toward the new building and plans began for the Dougherty Hospice House. Michael Dougherty, brother of long-time McKennan trustee Bill Dougherty, donated the money to honor his parents who died when he was only 15 and in memory of Bill's wife who, Michael noted, "was like a mother to me."[279] In addition, the Thomas M. Reardon Family Endowment contributed $500,000 toward an endowment fund for ongoing operating expenses. The 16-bed facility is larger than originally planned due to the outpouring of donations from the community, making it the largest hospice residence in the state of South Dakota.[280] The facility, which offers a warm, welcoming and homelike environment, is decorated with over 100 pieces of artwork from local artists. Dougherty House's walls are painted bright, warm shades and the rooms provide a variety of innovations to offer comfort, convenience and privacy.

The private rooms feature fireplaces, while the facility includes a small chapel, community rooms for large family gatherings, a kitchen area, garden and even a dog kennel for visitors to bring pets.

It was near the dog kennel that the late Bill Dougherty said he wanted to be if he ever needed hospice care; this was in order that he would have been near Higgins, his Maltese.[281] Dougherty, who donated $100,000 toward the Dougherty Hospice House, was a Sioux Falls businessman, lobbyist and former lieutenant governor.[282] A member of the Avera McKennan Board of Trustees from 1981-1997, he saw the hospital through the trying times of the 1980s when McKennan was challenged by low patient numbers and high debt to the more confident days of the 1990s when both the hospital's census and budget greatly improved. Invited to be on the board by Sister Colman Coakley, "his favorite person in the whole world," Dougherty felt that with regard to his work with McKennan Hospital, both the Dougherty Hospice House as well as the hospital's free clinic were the legacies for which he was most proud.[283]

In the early 1990s, Dougherty helped to establish the hospital's free clinic, known as the Avera McKennan Downtown Health Care Clinic.[284] He began this venture with the support of Sister Colman Coakley, Don Bierle, legal advisor to the Presentation and Benedictine Sisters in South Dakota and another McKennan trustee, Jeremiah Murphy. Murphy recalled that after a board meeting that focused on giving back to the community, the idea of a free clinic took root. First, they secured a building on 6th and Cliff for $200 per month and to help complete the process,

builders and contractors "donated time and materials. Plumbers, electricians and decorators all gave freely of their talents to transform a former fast food restaurant into a professional medical clinic."[285]

In October of 1992, the free clinic, welcoming persons without insurance, opened its doors and within months was serving hundreds of patients. It was soon clear that the need was quickly outpacing the clinic's space. Staff saw patients with problems as complex as Lou Gehrig's disease, Hodgkin's disease and cancer. In addition, the clinic welcomed patients from well beyond Sioux Falls—people from Minnesota and Iowa.

The numbers using the clinic continued to escalate and by the year 2000, over 5,000 persons a year arrived at the clinic's doors. That year the clinic moved to East 10th Street, a location that was twice the size of the Cliff Avenue clinic and offered three exam rooms with a fourth for procedures.[286] Within a few years the clinic again needed more space, and in 2007 it moved to its present location in downtown Sioux Falls.

Currently under the direction of Dr. James Barker and nurse Joanne Hindbjorgen, the clinic offers educational information, particularly on diabetes; does outreach work, including providing flu shots and other care; and has recently begun to offer psychiatric care one day per week. Hindbjorgen, a former Avera McKennan ER nurse, has been running the facility for 12 years. She notes that while the medical care is significant, the clinic provides an important social connection. "This is their clinic and we and the patients get to know each other on a first name basis... we are a breath of fresh air on the block."

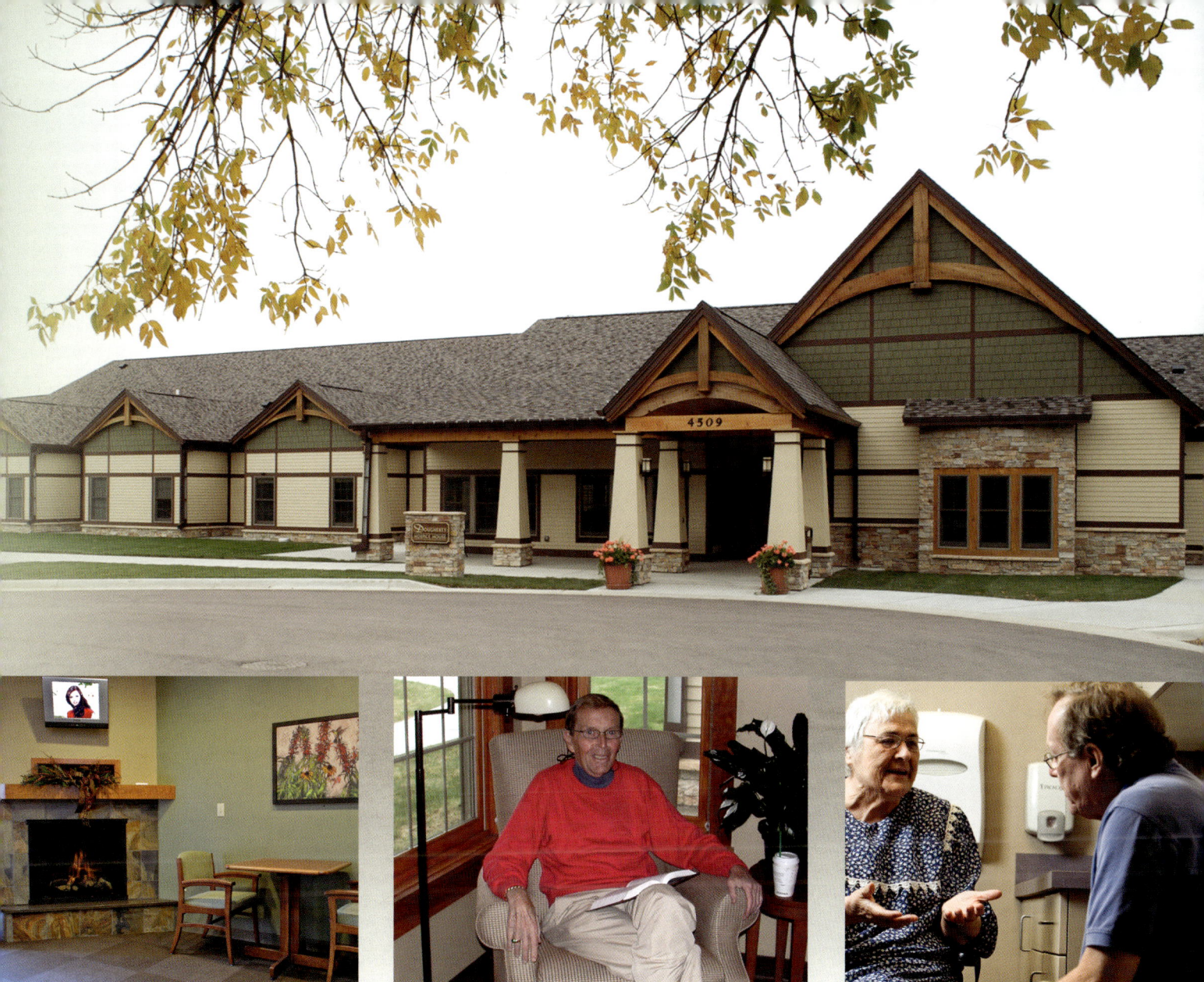

Bill Dougherty

Dr. James Barker

The numbers using the clinic continue to grow; it cared for over 5,800 persons in 2007 while during 2008-2009, the clinic handled over 8,500 patients.[287]

Supported by the hospital, the annual Great Tables Fundraiser and outside donations, the clinic relies on the help of many volunteers. In 1993 Bonnie Irvine, former supervisor of the clinic said: "The clinic couldn't operate without volunteers. Many are nursing or physician's assistant students" from local schools.[288] In 2006, USD medical students established the "Coyote Clinic," and with the help of volunteer doctors, it provides care one evening per month. Sister Mary Thomas, senior vice president of Mission Services, pointed out the important contribution made by the free clinic and its staff who, she stated, "have the compassion and can promote the dignity of the people who come…it is a very credible and public face of the mission in action." Now approaching its 20th year, Jeremiah Murphy reflected on the importance of the clinic: "It's a marvelous success…one of the things we agreed is that we would never brag about it. And we really don't. And I think—as my father always told me, 'The best publicity is what you get naturally.'"[289]

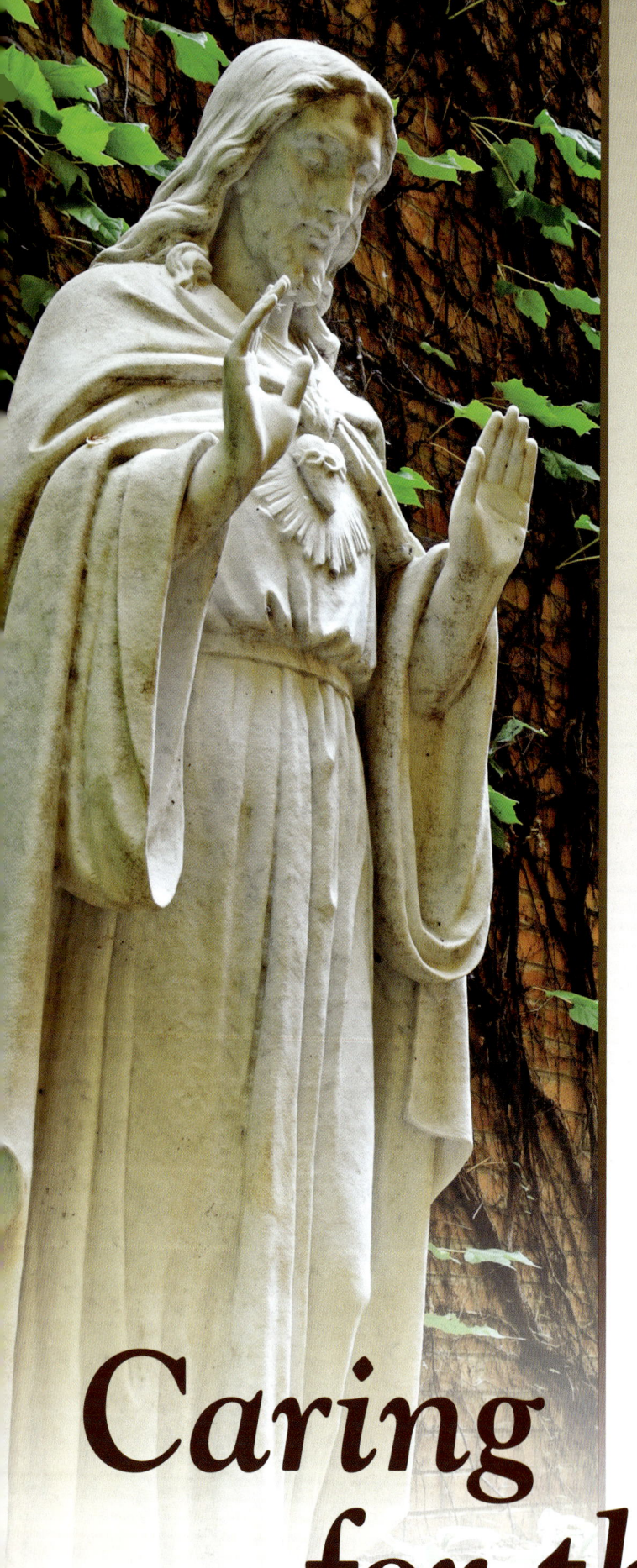

On the 50th anniversary of McKennan Hospital, the *Argus Leader* featured "A Minister's Views on Hospital Service" for which a Protestant minister, who desired to remain anonymous, reflected on how McKennan Hospital provided a community service. The minister wrote: "The hospital becomes the meeting ground for religion and medical science to attend to the basic needs of humanity" and, echoing Bishop O'Gorman's words from 50 years earlier, the minister observed that the hospital was a place for, "the doctor to attend the body and the minister or priest to attend the soul." The anonymous minister reflected on how the hospital becomes an extension of his parish and said that "the hospital has assumed part of the work of the church for the relief of human suffering." Thus, given that the hospital and the minister seek the same goal, he suggested that they search for opportunities of cooperation. "The hospital is more than a public institution, more than a public building. It is a spiritual lifeline where physical and spiritual needs of mankind are answered."[290]

This minister's comments would have pleased Helen McKennan who, as a devout Christian, expressed interest in having the hospital established with a Christian mission.[291] Since its inception, McKennan Hospital made clear that it offered its care to persons of all faiths. When it opened, McKennan Hospital had a full-time resident chaplain who, though a Catholic priest, was there to serve the spiritual needs of all the hospital's patients. Conveniently, the Roman

Caring for the Soul

Catholic Bishop's residence sat across from the hospital, and up until 1940 when it moved, the Bishop generally appointed his administrative assistant to be the hospital's chaplain. Of course, then as now, the Sisters provided spiritual care to the patients.

As the hospital grew, the demands upon pastoral care increased while the number of Sisters and priests decreased. In an effort to address this challenge, in 1968, the Presentation Order announced that in each of their hospitals they would create a department of pastoral care and by 1972 had begun the process of establishing a program that would offer Clinical Pastoral Education throughout the Presentation Health System. Called the Association for Clinical Pastoral Education (ACPE), this pastoral care training program has its roots in the early 20th century.[292] In 1973, McKennan Hospital next hired Father Lawrence Murtagh to provide training and education for local clergy of any denomination in order to improve the experience between pastor and patient. In 1974, the first six "graduates" completed the 30-week course which sought to make them "adept in ministering to the sick in hospitals, nursing homes and private homes." Each student, under the leadership of Fr. Murtagh, attended 14 hours of supervised learning per week, which included eight hours of making rounds with physicians.[293]

The *Argus Leader* interviewed some of the program's first graduates who discussed their experience and reflected on how their training helped them recognize that they needed to embrace both the process of living and dying personally and professionally. As one minister noted, prior to taking the course, he often went through a visit with a patient without ever talking about his or her feelings about death. "Now…somewhere along the line I ask, 'What do you think is going to happen?' That sort of opens up the door."

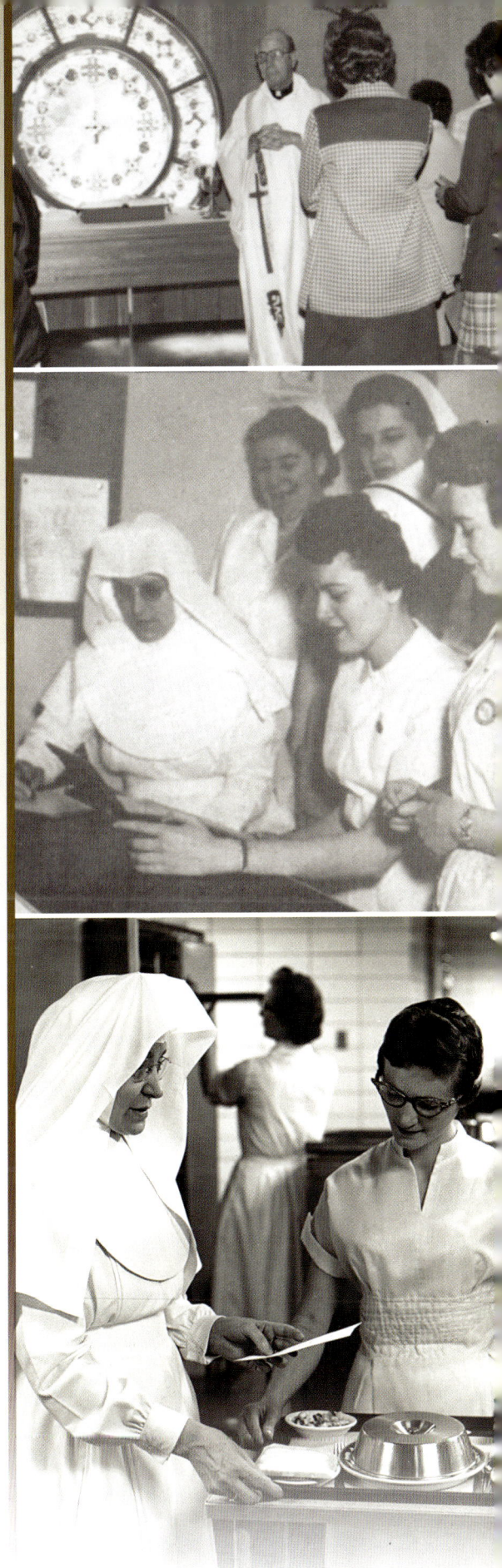

Another reflected that the program allowed him to recognize that when a member of his own congregation died, he too had the right to mourn:

> "I realized I was a human being who needed to grieve when someone close to me died. We (ministers) tend to see ourselves as a person who helps other people, encourages them to express their grief. We tend to see ourselves as the strong, supportive individual who can be emotionally detached."

This pastor noted that he came to realize that it was important that he too had the right to grieve the loss of a friend and should seek out others with whom he could share his feelings. After attending the program, these men helped the next set of incoming students learn how to minister to their flock during these most frightening and challenging of times.[294]

In 1981 Rev. Peter Holland, a United Church of Christ minister, became director of what had formally become a Clinical Pastoral Education program.[295] The late Fr. Murtagh continued to teach in the program—as both he and Holland were certified by the National Association for Clinical Pastoral Education. By 1991, some 350 students had completed the CPE program.

In 1992 the Rev. Steven P. Corum joined the staff and he and Holland teach courses throughout the region. While the majority of students are either ministers or seminary students, CPE has also welcomed nurses, doctors and others over the years. To the present, the Avera Clinical Pastoral Education Center has trained some 1,500 students–including some who seek to become certified as supervisors in CPE.

Of the program Holland reflected, "You and the person you're working with are changed. Both people have to be open to the spirit."[296]

To the present, hospital chaplains reach out to all areas. Clara Johnson, director of Trauma, EMS Education, Chaplaincy and Bariatric Services, summarized the integral role that Avera McKennan's chaplains play: "There is a chaplain that responds to every death in the house–24/7–to every trauma team and every Code Blue, as well as palliative medicine meetings, multidisciplinary meetings, meeting with patients and families in the Emergency Department or in the intensive care units, making rounds on the regular units—always, always with the goal that they bring a presence of Christ. They walk with people and families who are in their most critical, painful times—the death of a child or a spouse—whatever that might be. There's no fixing it but to listen and to be there. There is no proselytizing, no evangelism... The chaplains listen to others, wherever they are."[297]

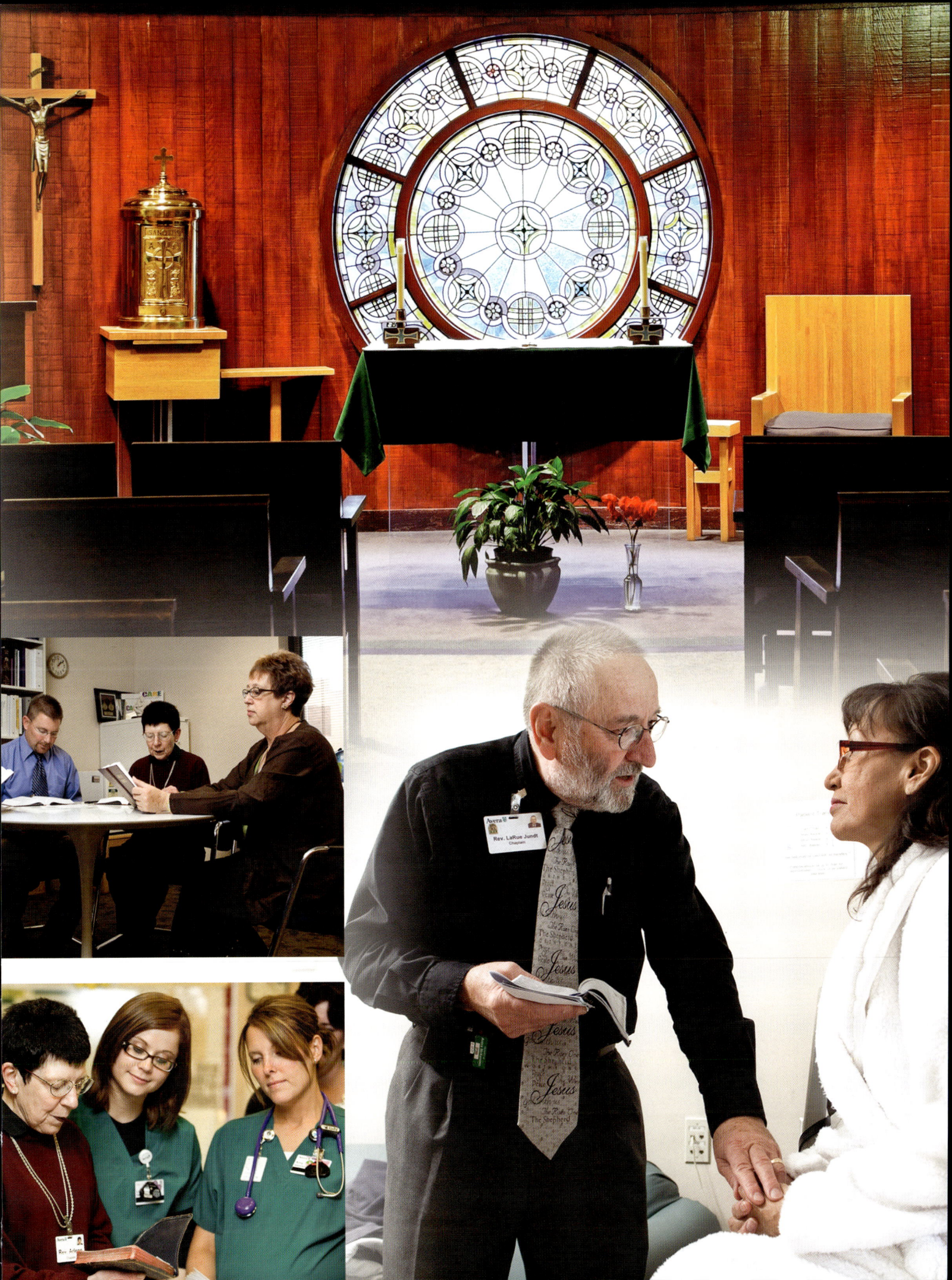

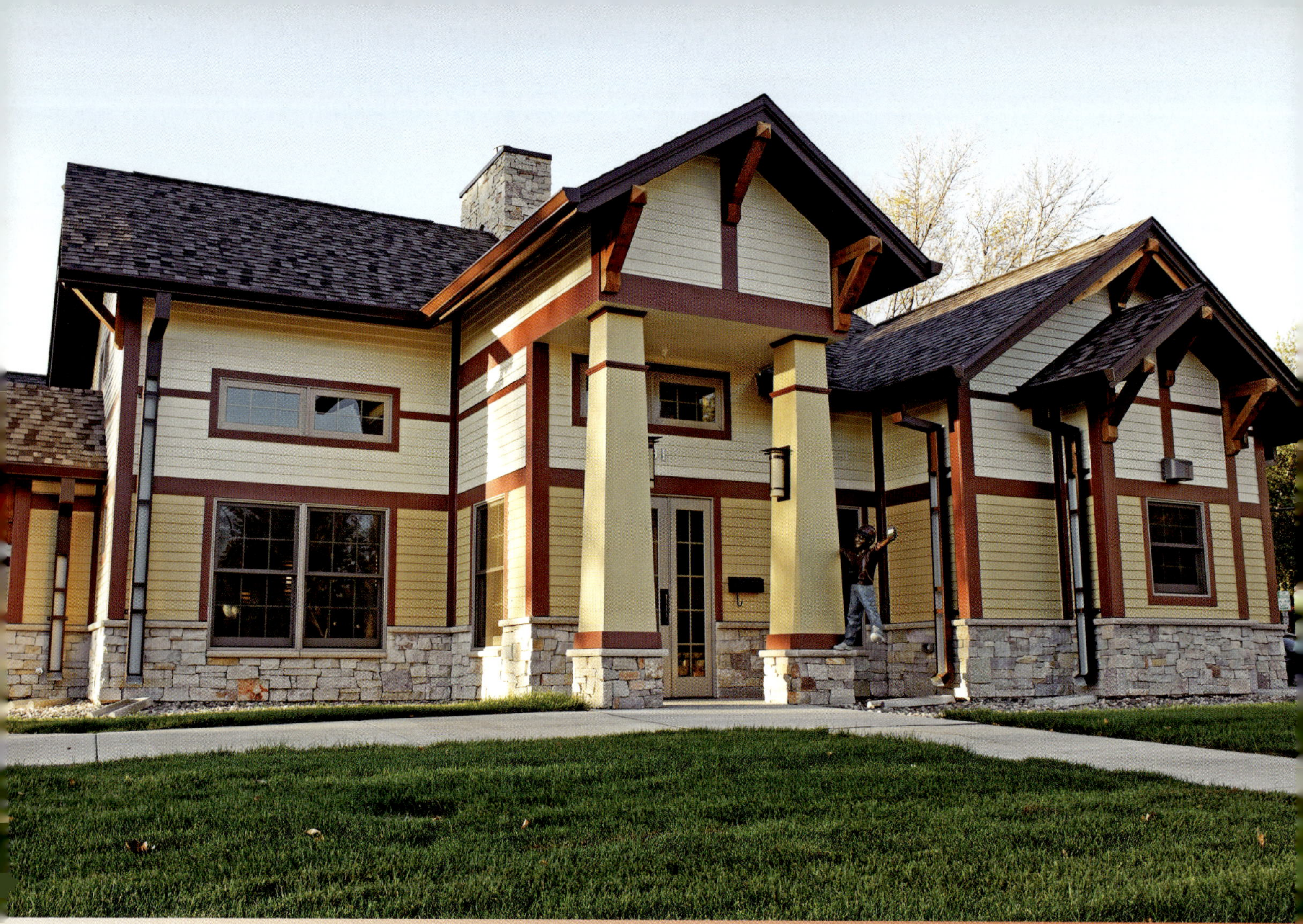

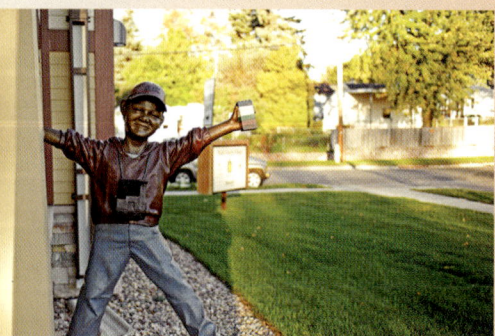

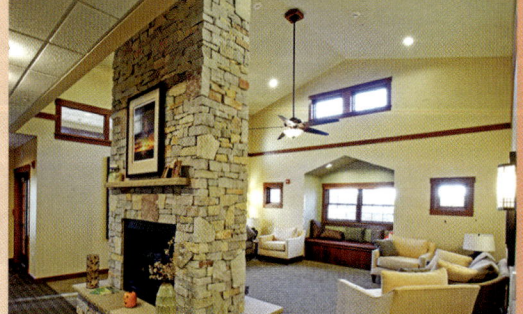

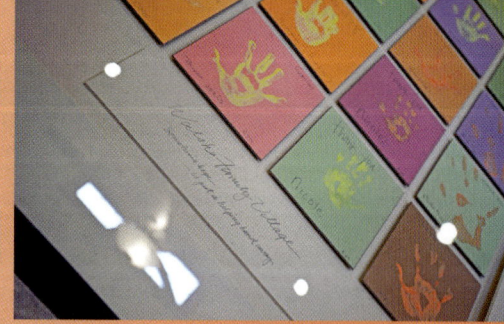

Of the many patients from around the world that McKennan has helped, a young boy named Carlos Antonio Vasquez Hernandes from Los Cabos, Mexico particularly touched the hearts of many. Tom Walsh, founder of the Los Cabos Children's Foundation, brought Carlos to Sioux Falls in order for Carlos to receive treatment for his leukemia. During his months in Sioux Falls, Avera McKennan and the local community welcomed Carlos and his family. Tragically Carlos lost his battle with cancer in 2003; nevertheless, he became an inspiration to "all those he met to reach out and help the children in need in Los Cabos."

On August 11, 2008, the Walsh Family Village, which is host to the Casa de Carlitos Welcome Center, Nano Nagle Inn and the Ronald McDonald House opened; already every room was reserved by a family that needed accommodation while a loved one received treatment at Avera McKennan.[298] The village was funded entirely by donations and, most notably, a $1.5 million gift from Tom and Kathy Walsh and the Los Cabos Children's Foundation. At the entrance of the Casa de Carlitos Welcome Center and swinging from a support column, just as any curious child would, is young Carlos with a smile on his face and Lego in one hand. This is a sculpture of Carlos whose "spirit and depth of understanding of life was very profound for a 7-year-old." The sculpture, commissioned by the Avera McKennan Foundation in appreciation of the gift from Tom and Kathy Walsh and the Los Cabos Children's Foundation, is the creation of Darwin Wolf,

The Walsh Family Village is just one example of how Avera McKennan has sought to extend care to the greater community. Dolores Harrington, author of *A Woman's Will…A Sister's Way: The McKennan Hospital Story,* which looked at the hospital's first 50 years, noted that from the start the hospital's kitchen was always busy—feeding persons both in and outside of the hospital. First run by Sister Magdalen Murphy, the kitchen prepared meals for patients and employees. In addition, noted Harrington, "migrant workers and down-on-their-luck transients of varying types who wandered across the nation" gravitated to Sister Magdalen's kitchen. Sister Magdalen, according to Sister Rose McCormick, would refer to these persons as her "relatives" and never hesitated to provide them with a meal. The provision of food out the back of the cafeteria continued though, as Harrington wrote, when a group of five paid 75 cents for a cab to get

Giving Back…

an award-winning sculptor.[299] Wolf said that Carlos even inspired him; just before Wolf received his commission he fell from a roof that he was shingling and broke his back and leg. Wolf used the sculpting of Carlos' statue to get him back on his feet. Wolf wanted Carlos to look as if he had "a touch of rambunctious rebellion" welcoming all comers to his house and looking for a friend with whom to play.[300]

them to McKennan for a free meal, Sister Bonaventure Hoffman, the hospital administrator at the time stated: "I'll tell you right now…we put them to work before we fed them!"[301]

In another example, McKennan Hospital offered what today we would call long-term care to a few elderly patients. Dr. Russell Orr recalled that in the days

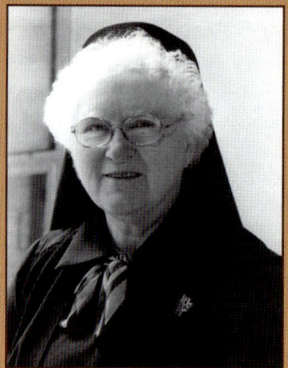

Sister Bonaventure
Hoffman

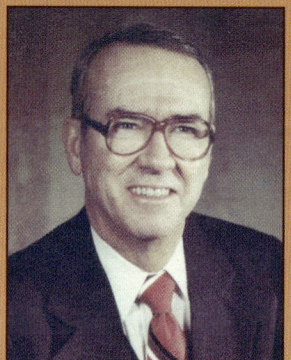

Dr. Russell Orr

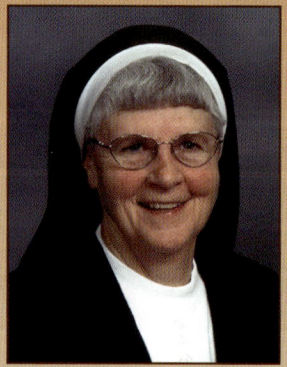

Sister Roch Whittaker

before Social Security the hospital housed elderly patients for the long term, and among them was his wife's uncle—Mr. Patrick Burke from Ireland:

"He was a patient there, and he was one of the type of patients without any source of income. The nuns would accept him without any guarantee of payment of anything. There was a basement area in which they had large rooms in which four beds could easily fit, and there weren't any screens between them or shades or anything, but these were male patients, and they'd be cared for as long as necessary."[302]

Over the years McKennan Hospital has sought other ways to give back to the community and, beginning in the 1980s and running for approximately 10 years, the hospital offered a Christmas dinner for those who would be alone for the holiday. Having been organized under the auspices of Sister Roch Whittaker, director of Mission Effectiveness, hospital volunteers, staff and their families served those who attended. Linda Olson, marketing specialist and an Avera McKennan employee since 1977, remembered the Christmas dinners and how "Sister Roch…put all of that together. And we had quite a team." The hospital sent vans out to pick up persons who did not have transportation. As Olson recalled, "Back then, of course, we didn't have cell phones. We all had walkie-talkies and we would have a group at the hospital who would relay, 'We have somebody for you to pick up.' They would bring them to the hospital and we had people there to greet them, to coat check, get them through the cafeteria line and get them food. The whole hospital was involved with that, and it was really a nice event."[303] Of the Christmas dinner the *Argus Leader* reported, "In many cases, those eating dinner at McKennan would have eaten their Christmas meal alone."[304] By 1991, the Christmas dinner had grown to something beyond just a meal as McKennan employees added to the season by collecting donations of food, clothing and gifts to give to a number of local charities. In 1992, the hospital was host to over 350 people at the dinner.[305]

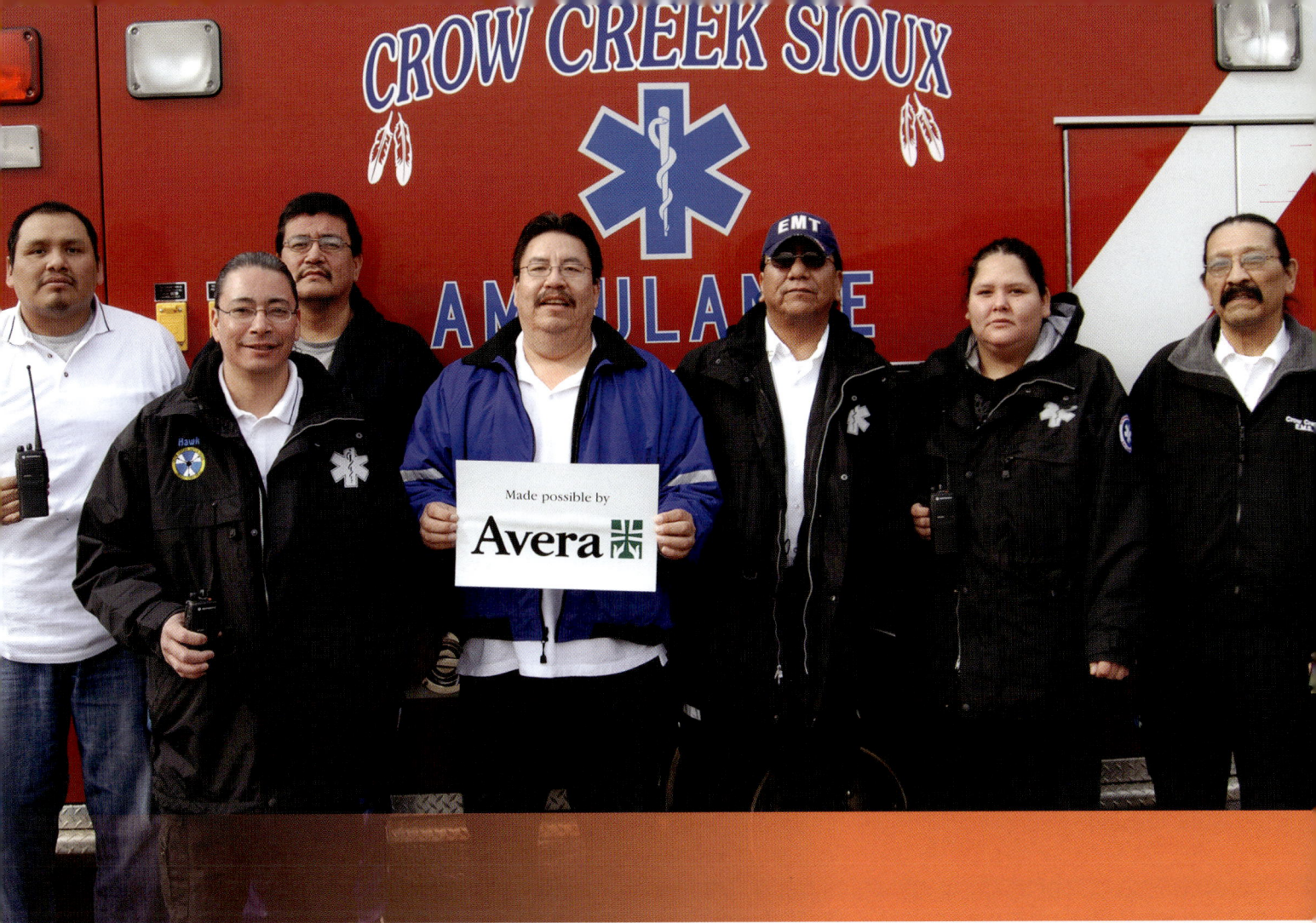

In a more contemporary example, Avera McKennan has developed relationships with Lower Brule and Crow Creek Indian Reservations. As a result of reduced federal funding, it became clear that the two tribes were in serious need of basic medical equipment including wheelchairs, walkers and crutches. Thus, both Avera McKennan and Avera Home Medical Equipment now provide gently used equipment to the tribes. In 2008, a grant through Avera Health supplied Crow Creek with a much needed ambulance and uniforms for the EMTs who work for the service. Lower Brule had a matching grant from the Shakopee tribe, and thus in this case, Avera offered financial support. Fred Slunecka stated: "Our promise to [the tribes] was that whatever we did would be reliable and long

standing." The hope now is to also integrate the tribes into Avera McKennan's *e*CARE network.[306]

There are many other examples of how Avera McKennan cares for the community. John Hughes, chair of McKennan's Board of Trustees (1989-1992), reflected on the role of the sisters not just in running of the hospital but in caring for those beyond the hospital walls. He remembered that during board meetings when trustees found themselves deeply engaged in discussion about the various business needs of the hospital, eventually one of the sisters would stop the meeting and remind them of the mission: "to care for God's people and to be fair to our employees."[307]

Ambassadors, Pink Ladies, Candy Stripers, Red Jackets and MEN

In the tradition of Helen McKennan who, before giving away her treasure may well have volunteered her time for the care for persons in her community, Avera McKennan Hospital & University Health Center has quietly been aided by many volunteers who, early in the hospital's existence, formed the Hospital's Auxiliary. Established in 1936 by the wives of McKennan doctors, at their first meeting the group determined that "each lady was asked to contact four others and bring them to the next meeting." The ladies then began to meet on the second Monday of each month and after a "dessert luncheon, served by the sisters, [the women spent] the afternoon in sewing for the hospital."[308]

Not long after its inception, the Auxiliary began to raise funds for the hospital. It decided to sponsor an annual charity ball, "proceeds of which were to be used for hospital equipment;" and these first charitable balls raised between $3,000 and $5,000 annually. The money went toward everything from the more mundane of an ice cream machine, coffee and tea pots for various areas to the more relevant including two oxygen analyzers for obstetrics and an Iron Lung for the hospital. In 1945, for example, the Auxiliary "gave $3,500 for kitchen equipment and $200 for the Student Loan Fund." All of this was raised by an Auxiliary with over 300 members.[309]

In the post-war years, the annual charity ball continued to bring benefits to the hospital. In 1950, for example, monies from the ball bought a new vacillator bed and a fully equipped bacteriological laboratory; three years later the Auxiliary helped the hospital buy one of the area's first Isolette Infant Incubators; in 1955 the charity ball's earnings provided a newly renovated student lounge in St. Mary's Hall and in 1960 the Auxiliary purchased a Circolectric bed for the hospital.[310] "April in Paris" was the theme for the ball held on April 27, 1962, with invitations sent to over 1,000 persons in the area and, after dancing, the ball featured a midnight breakfast. The event went on to yield almost $10,000, and the hospital spent the money to remodel "the occupational therapy department, the therapy unit and the sundeck in the psychiatric unit of the hospital."[311]

The hospital ball continued over the years with the 1989 Auxiliary's charity ball breaking all records by bringing in over $17,000. "This is the best ever!" exclaimed Sister Colman Coakley. The money went toward the purchase of new equipment at the McKennan Childbirth Center Intensive Care Nursery, including warmers, ventilators and bed scales.

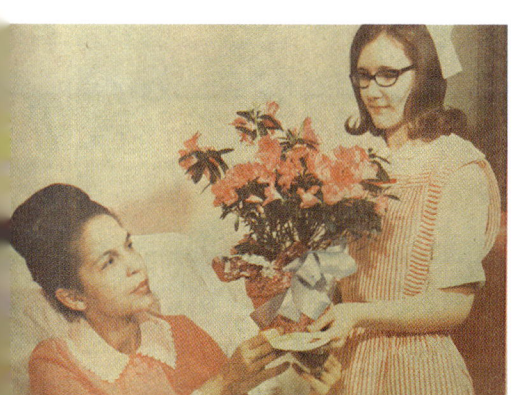
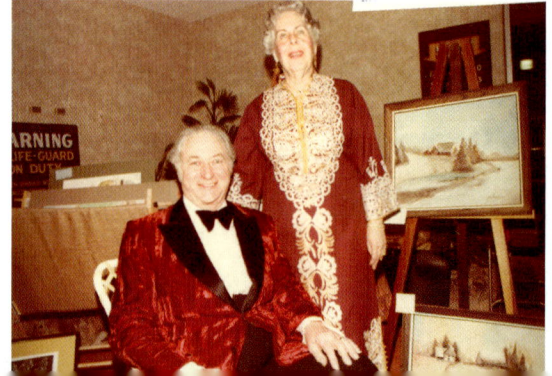
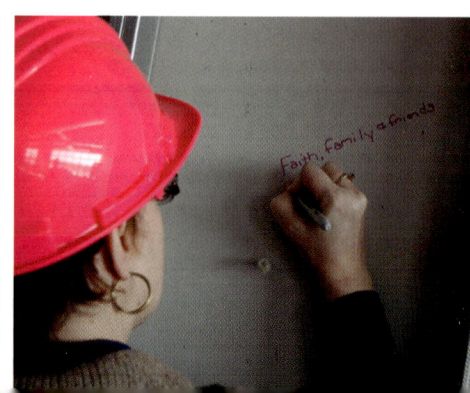

The ball's theme was "Orientale" and over 300 persons attended. Surpassing the previous year's donation by over $2,000, this overwhelming support was an important recognition by the community.

Over the years, the Auxiliary also sought to "serve as an ally of the hospital in public relations and volunteer service." In 1961, McKennan was the first hospital in the state to host Candy Stripers and by 1962 the hospital had 83 teenagers volunteering; that year *Parents Magazine* awarded the group its annual "youth group achievement awards." Candy Stripers, a national organization founded in 1942, was composed of female teenagers who volunteered their time doing various tasks, including helping "in the linen room, conduct[ing] messenger service, minor laboratory work and entertain[ing] in pediatrics." This program sought to encourage a sense of civic responsibility and was another way to introduce teenagers to the possibility of a future in health care. Populating one-third of the nation's hospitals, these teenagers dressed in "gay red and white striped pinafores" were an added support to McKennan Hospital's "pink ladies." [312] Called such because of their pink smocks, the "pink ladies'" motto was "continuous service and always with the same pleasant smile, a kind word and a helping hand," as noted by the *Argus Leader* in 1961. Long-time hospital employee Betty Elkjer, who worked as a secretary to Sister Bonaventure Hoffman, helped to start McKennan Hospital's "pink ladies," as well as bring on board the Candy Stripers, and the Red Coats, young men who worked as volunteers.[313]

While the Auxiliary, Pink Ladies, Red Coats and Candy Stripers steadily offered their time and talents to the hospital, other than the Red Coats, these groups were comprised of females. However, in 1986 the *Argus Leader* recognized that McKennan had begun to welcome adult male volunteers to the hospital. The McKennan Escort Network (MEN) began in November of 1986 with 20 volunteers chaperoning patients throughout the hospital. For four hours one or two days per week, these men helped patients and visitors find where they needed to be in the hospital. To the present, Avera McKennan is helped by over 1,000 volunteers, with at least 20 percent of them being men.

In 2007, long after the annual balls had ceased, the Auxiliary changed its name to Ambassadors, but this did not mean that the good work of those who so generously give of their time and talent came to an end. In 2009, over 80 persons volunteered every day at Avera McKennan, the equivalent of almost 45 full-time hospital employees. Volunteer Bill Butler, retired from John Morrell & Co., may have summed it up best when he said, "What you do for somebody else, they say comes back two fold…we're supposed to be our brother's keeper and help each other." [314]

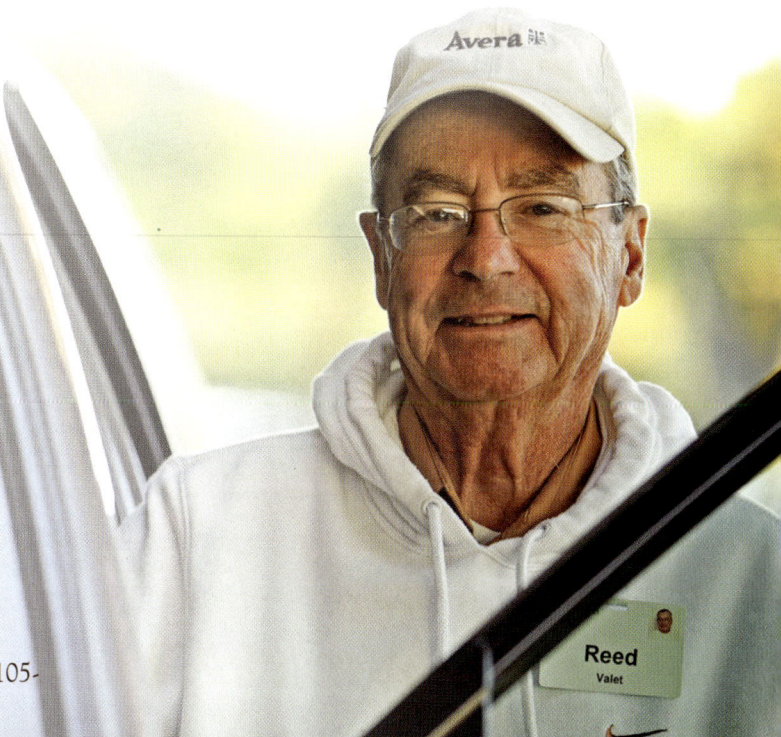

Looking to the Future

When McKennan Hospital opened in 1911 it was a state-of-the-art medical facility – a sanitary environment in which patients could receive superior care. A century later, Avera McKennan Hospital & University Health Center remains on the cutting edge of health care.

Now, not only a hospital, Avera McKennan is an integrated care network of regional hospitals, clinics, long-term care facilities and more. Avera McKennan provides an array of 60 medical specialties, some of which are not offered elsewhere in the region, such as hepatology. In 2007, the Avera Center for Liver Disease opened – the first specialty clinic for diseases of the liver in the state of South Dakota. Avera McKennan recently added the subspecialty of women's care known as urogynecology, and has the region's only fellowship-trained urogynecologist. Avera McKennan is also proud to offer state-of-the-art technology. The new Avera Cancer Institute houses some of the latest technology for cancer care, available at only a few locations in the United States. Surgical robotics allows surgeons to offer minimally invasive procedures that translate into less pain, less blood loss and a shorter recovery time for patients.

In the past, treating illness or injury was the job of the lone physician, and the hospital simply served as a place for doctors to practice their art of healing. Today, health care is a collaborative effort of a multidisciplinary team including primary and specialty care physicians, physician assistants and nurse practitioners, nurses, social workers, pharmacists, therapists, technicians, lab scientists and chaplains to name just a few. While health systems continue to pursue cures for disease, they have come to realize that it is just as important to promote healthy living and preventative medicine in order to keep disease from happening in the first place.

In the century to come, Avera will mobilize its resources in a collaborative effort to meet the coming challenges, including national health care reform. Avera is uniquely positioned for health care reform, one aspect of which is a changed focus from making people well to keeping people well. Through its sense of mission and health ministry, Avera McKennan has long advocated care and concern for the whole person – body, mind and spirit, and will continue to build on this model. Another aspect of health care reform is integration of services. Avera has established a comprehensive network of facilities across the upper Midwest, and at the same time has successfully integrated numerous physicians into the organization. Avera has been at the forefront of technological advancements that bring specialized medical services to rural areas, through innovations such as telemedicine, eICU and eEmergency.

It all started over 100 years ago with Helen Gale McKennan's dream of a community hospital that would serve and benefit humanity. Her dream became reality through a group of dedicated women, who, over the years, have gathered around them a vast array of expertise, talent and ability. Yet, the Sisters of the Presentation and Benedictine Orders have also maintained that health care cannot be successfully provided unless it is driven by a mission which is rooted in the healing ministry of Jesus.

In 1997 Bob Voglewede, Vice President for Mission Services with Avera Health, reflected upon the spirit of the Sisters within the greater health system and noted that there "is something special…a special spirit. Without them we wouldn't be who we are." Voglewede then asked what might happen if the Sisters disappear…where will we be? In 2010, Avera McKennan hospitalist Dr. Jennifer McKay offered a reassuring answer to Voglewede's question:

 "As long as we keep our mission in front of us, we're always going to be able to change and adapt, exceed expectations and set standards. I'm honestly not worried about the future. Every time we ask the question, 'How does this make something better for our patients?' everything falls into place. That's what God asks us to do; that's why the Sisters are here; that's why we exist. Everything that's happening around us is just a reflection of that."[315]

Dr. McKay's words express the legacy established by the Sisters of the Presentation of the Blessed Virgin Mary 100 years ago. Despite their diminished numbers, they continue to ensure that what remains is the mission they established when they opened McKennan Hospital on December 17, 1911.

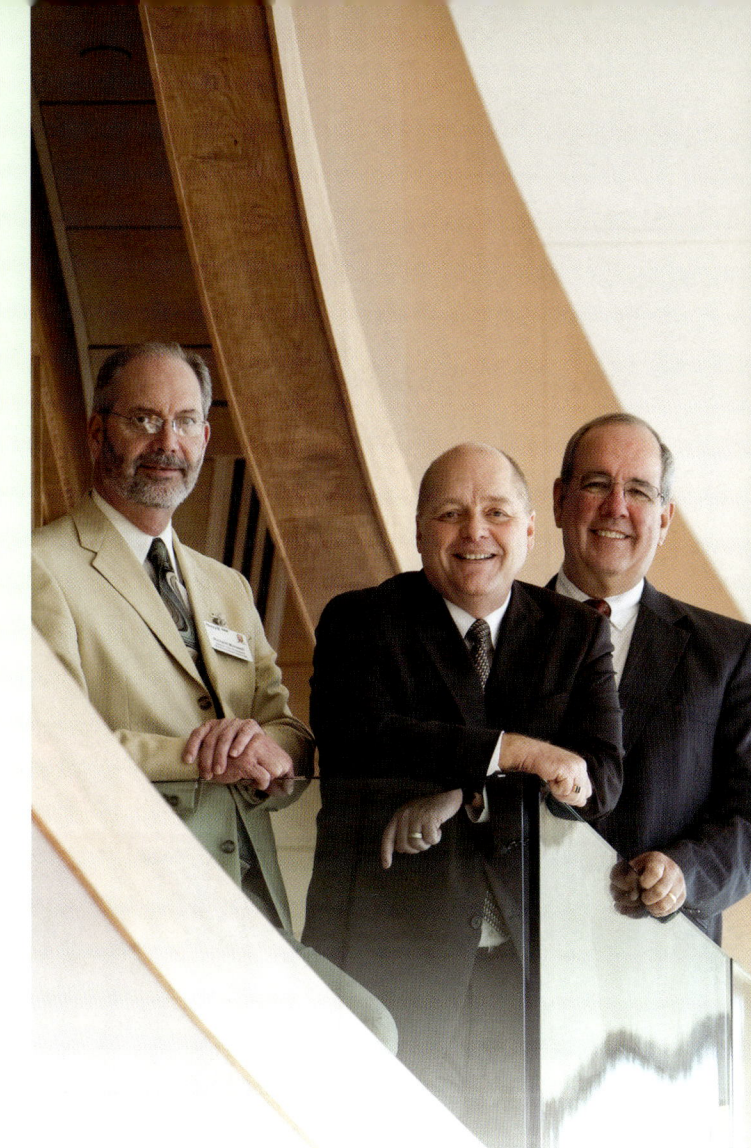

Richard Molseed, Senior Vice President of Environmental Services; Fred Slunecka, Avera Health Chief Operating Officer and Dr. Dave Kapaska, Regional President Avera McKennan Hospital & University Health Center

While medicine becomes more complex and technologically advanced, the mission statement of Avera McKennan remains a simple but timeless message that, if adhered to, will allow the health system to move forward with integrity:

Avera is a health ministry rooted in the Gospel. Our mission is to make a positive impact in the lives and health of persons and communities by providing quality services guided by Christian values.

Remembering the 1910s-1920s

Dr. T.J. Billion Jr. grew up on 21st Street and clearly recalls the Sisters—always in pairs—walking down the boulevard for their evening exercise. With the other neighborhood kids, he was a frequent visitor to the kitchen in the basement of the hospital. "The nuns always had bananas and cookies for us," recalled Billion. "They were special cookies with a big piece of marshmallow on top and covered with white frosting." "McKennan Hospital: Expanding to Serve a Growing Community." Kathleen McGreevy, *All of Us*, July 1992.

Remembering the 1930s

"We were all aware of the [poor economic] condition of the country at that time. The hospital obtained its main source of vegetables from a farm they had, which…probably [sat] where the zoo is. They would bring in fresh vegetables daily. And, of course, they had their own bakery." Kathleen McGreevy, "Interview with **Dorcas Baldwin**," January, 2006.

"They had a wire contraption in the form of a half circle that was put over the bed. A blanket was put over this. We heated a kettle of solution on our stove in the kitchen until it was dangerous to handle. We put it in this electric Crockpot-thing, plugged it in, and that created steam in a hose that went under this blanket. There was medication in the solution, and [patients] were to receive these steam treatments many times a day. They complained bitterly, but it was given to them. So that was one way of [treating] pneumonia." Kathleen McGreevy, "Interview with **Dorcas Baldwin**," January, 2006.

Remembering the 1940s-1950s

"In the 1940s, the medical records department was in the old building, the original hospital building. There were two rooms. Sister Ursula had one room, and I was in the next room. All the records were kept around the shelves and in file cabinets and so forth. I didn't even have a desk; I had a library table. And the records were kept, the admissions and discharges, in big ledgers. Everything was handwritten, except the dictation from the doctors, which was typed." Kathleen McGreevy, "Interview with **Madonna Clark**," March 23, 2006.

"It was approaching Christmas and the Sisters] really needed a car. We mentioned it to Dr. Donahoe and he said, 'You take care of the employee part, and we'll take care of the doctors.' This was during the war years, when cars were difficult to get.

"When the Sisters were having their Christmas party, Dr. Stuart Grove, who was the chief of staff at that time, went down to the dining area where they were having the party, and he knocked at the door, and one of the Sisters came over. Right away she started to close the door, because they were having their little party, and they didn't think the doctors would approve of something like that. But he put his foot in the door, went in and presented them with the keys to the car. They were dumbfounded, to say the least.

"Several weeks later, over the loud-speaking system, came an announcement: 'Will someone please go to the ambulance drive! There's a blue baby there.' So they went to the ambulance drive, and the blue baby was the new car." Kathleen McGreevy, "Interview with **Madonna Clark**," March 23, 2006.

"One day I was coming out of the chapel, and Sister Monica said, 'Madonna, I found a pair of gloves in the chapel. Did you happen to lose yours?' And I said, 'No, Sister, I didn't.' She said, 'What size do you wear?' And I told her. When we had our Christmas party, held in what was originally the Bishop's residence, all the department heads who were ladies got white doeskin gloves. The Sisters used to go into Chicago on a buying trip before Christmas, and that's why she was asking the size of the gloves. Nobody could give a party like the nuns. Nobody. And they gave us beautiful things. I still have a pair of pillowcases that Sister David did all this filled-in stitching on. They always did those things for us. There wasn't an eight-hour day in those days. You worked till all was done. You didn't get overtime pay. But when you got ready to go on vacation, you'd maybe find an envelope on your desk with an old note. I remember I got one from Mother Cornelia. 'This doesn't begin to make up the overtime pay for all the hours you've put in, but maybe it'll give you a little extra spending money on your vacation,' she wrote." Kathleen McGreevy, "Interview with **Madonna Clark**," March 23, 2006.

"Sister Ligouri was in charge of the chapel…took care of the altars and everything. She was just the most saintly person and so very, very kind, very capable. She would go with the priest to take the Blessed Sacrament to the patients. Sister Berchmans was in dietary, and she was in charge of the visitors' dining room for all the doctors and priests and so forth. And, oh, how she would wait on them and see that they had everything at their disposal. They were just wonderful, wonderful women." Kathleen McGreevy, "Interview with **Madonna Clark**," March 23, 2006.

Remembering the 1950s-1960s

"We had no TVs in the hospital when I came in 1952, and when TV started coming into its own, the Auxiliary took it as a project. Mrs. Dunn would roll them around to the patients' rooms on a cart. If a patient wanted a TV, they charged them something. When we built the 1958 building, that had all the magic of the time. It had all private rooms, and they were equipped with TVs. People wanted more - they wanted a private room; they wanted bathrooms. In the old building we had two bathrooms on one floor…. All these [new] things added to the cost." Kathleen McGreevy, "Interview with **Sister Colman Coakley**," February 23, 2006.

"Sister Camillus Shealy was also from Ireland. She had many, many friends in Sioux Falls. When we built the 1958 building, she was nursing supervisor on what we then called One North, which was a medical floor. It was the latest in technology then. And Sister Camillus loved it and guarded the rooms and made sure that the doctors knew when there were rooms available. Employees loved her. When the carts came up with the patient trays, the nurses used to laugh and say no matter what they were doing, they had to drop it because Sister Camillus would go out in the middle of the hall and say, "Trays, girls, trays," so that they had to leave everything and get the trays out to the patients with the food. Kathleen McGreevy, "Interview with **Sister Colman Coakley**," February 23, 2006.

"I spent 45 years at McKennan and the Presentation Health System. I came to McKennan in 1952, when the campus included only the 1911 and the 1919 buildings. You approached the front door of the hospital [and had to go] up about eight to 10 steps. In that day, 'handicap accessible' was not a concept." Kathleen McGreevy, Russell McKnight and Margaret Preston "Interview with **Sister Colman Coakley**," September 30, 2008.

"People would ask, 'Well, where did the sisters live?' In the very early days, they lived up on the fourth floor of the 1919 Building, and the nurses lived up there, too. But when I came to McKennan, there was the basement of the 1911 Building, the west end of it. We had several rooms and a community room down there, and that was about the extent of it, but that's where we lived." Kathleen McGreevy, Russell McKnight and Margaret Preston "Interview with **Sister Colman Coakley**," September 30, 2008.

"The dedication on the medical staff was an example for all of us. I recall a bad blizzard in the late 1950s. Traffic was at a halt in the city. Doctors and employees were snowbound. Only the ambulances were out that day. The snow was piled as high as the front door of the 1958 building…. Dr. Verlynne Volin was the only doctor at the hospital that morning, and he stayed all day and all night and delivered the OB patients. I was the only one in the office that morning because the other employees couldn't get to work." Kathleen McGreevy, Russell McKnight and Margaret Preston "Interview with **Sister Colman Coakley**," September 30, 2008.

"In the 1960s, one of the biggest surprises to me at McKennan was the ceremony when the priests would bring communion [to] the patients. A Sister would precede the priest, and they would ring a little bell, and if they were on the elevator going from here to there no one else could get on at the same time. I'm a Lutheran and that was very, very foreign to me." Kathleen McGreevy, "Interview with **Dr. Loren Amundson**," June 23, 2008.

"Shortly after I got here in 1966, I felt that we needed nuclear imaging in Sioux Falls. Nobody was doing that, and the potential for good diagnosis with radionucleids was taking off. At that time, we could get licensed by the Atomic Energy Commission, now the Nuclear Regulatory Commission, because you had to have a federal license to handle the radionucleids. So I went and got on-site training. We had one gamma camera, which was a very primitive instrument at that time. It had one crystal and as things developed we got multiple-crystal cameras. We got computer tomography. A whole bevy of nuclear imaging tests came along, so that we developed the Nuclear Medicine Department at the hospital." Kathleen McGreevy, "Interview with **Dr. Loyd Wagner**," October 20, 2008.

"I was very intimidated by the Sisters, not having grown up with any in our little town of Spencer. I was doing clinicals and assigned to One North where Sister Camillus was the head nurse. Just a little bit of a lady from Ireland. She was excellent at starting IVs, which were done with only a straight needle at that time. She took me with her and said 'you pray girlie, while I stick.' A few days later she took me with her and said: 'You stick girlie, I will pray.' Fortunately for the patient her prayer was answered. After that she would just send me on my own." Kathleen McGreevy, "E-mail Correspondence with **LaVonne Gaspar**," December 10, 2009.

Remembering the 1970s-1990s

"Well, up until probably about five years ago, you had to be in complete uniform and that [included a] cap. There were no slacks, it was all dress uniforms. Then when these pantsuits started coming out, they wore those and then they got away from wearing their hats, as long as they had their identification with their pins. I think the older nurses really felt a loss because you weren't going to work if you didn't have your cap on. Everyone had a different cap and different pins. Then you had a stripe on the side [of the cap during] your junior year. Your senior year, you had two stripes on the side. After you graduated you had one black stripe across the cap." Susan Peterson, "Interview with **Lillian Arends**," June 29, 1978.

"Don Bierle was on the original Health Care Council of the Presentation Sisters, and he was on the McKennan Board of Directors for many years. He was legal counsel. He was a moving force in our health care ministry. He also was very active in the South Dakota legislature. Well, you know, Don Bierle was a go-getter. He could make decisions. He was the force behind and led the way to get the Health and Education Facilities Authority. That's where we get the tax-exempt bonds. He was also on the South Dakota Housing Authority. He was a co-founder of the American Academy of Hospital Attorneys. And he was also much into sports. I think he got the Hall of Fame for the sports going. I mean, he was interested in everything. You just wonder how he had the time do everything, but he had an enormous capacity for absorbing things and getting things done." Kathleen McGreevy, "Interview with **Sister Colman Coakley**," February 23, 2006 and Kathleen McGreevy and Margaret Preston "Interview with **Sister Colman Coakley**," January 30, 2009.

"The social services department at McKennan was the first one in South Dakota, and I really thought the Sisters were forward-thinking in realizing that, in addition to the physical and spiritual needs of patients that were being met, that there were some emotional and psychological needs that patients had. Some of the physicians thought it was unnecessary, but my biggest champion was Dr. Lynn DeMarco. He could see that his patients could use that kind of service, and he did a lot toward helping other doctors see that there was a place for social work in the hospital." Kathleen McGreevy, "Interview with **Sandra Rockafellow**," July 20, 2006.

"We held the doctors appreciation party around St. Patrick's Day and the employees appreciation party around Christmas time. Because we had fewer employees we'd give each employee a gift. The doctors loved those parties, and to this day if I see Dr. Loren Amundson, he talks about the parties." Kathleen McGreevy, "Interview with **Sister Colman Coakley**," February 23, 2006

"Everyone knew Sister David Dorn. She'd come up from the laundry, which was in the basement, wearing her full habit and high-top tennis shoes. She had some foot problems and those high-tops were the only shoes she could find that were comfortable." Kathleen McGreevy, "Interview with **Fred Slunecka**," February 11, 2010.

"Well, I think you always have to look at how much money you're borrowing… Do you have the capability of paying it back? Those were the decisions that the board had to make. [We would] say, 'Well, we're meeting the needs of people. If it's God's work, it'll work out,' and the Sisters had faith in God and trust, and then, with the advice of these board members, we felt we had the capability of paying it back. But there were times you just squirmed when you heard the big amounts of money that were placed in front of the board to make decisions on. Like I said, you have to take a risk if you're going to serve people." Kathleen McGreevy, Russell McKnight and Margaret Preston "Interview with **Sister Colman Coakley**," September 30, 2008.

"I think that the [Presentation Health System] corporate board wanted to be able to get bonding for not only McKennan Hospital but also the other [Presentation] hospitals…. And these places were having a hard time getting funding to build new buildings because they were small hospitals. Sometimes their financial statements weren't very good, so they could maybe get bonding, but they'd have to pay real high interest rates because of that.

"So the corporate board wanted to get what they called a master trust indenture, and they used the financial statements of all the hospitals, and they put all the financial statements together, and all of a sudden it would be a much bigger pie, much bigger revenues and much bigger profits. It was very controversial, because we were using our financials [and] we would have to guarantee these bonds, even though they were facilities that our board had no control over.

"But in the final vote the McKennan board voted to join this master trust indenture. But I'm sure that the master trust indenture as a whole was good. It enabled all these hospitals, like St. Luke's and Mitchell to build new buildings and get real favorable interest rates that they wouldn't have had if we didn't do it. Kathleen McGreevy, "Interview with **Paul Connelly**," December 17, 2007.

"We are very committed to rural health care, and I think since we've become involved in a number of the rural communities that health care has been strengthened tremendously in those communities. We've been able to help them build hospitals, get new equipment, recruit the leaders, and provide benefits and salary to staff in a way that they maybe couldn't have if they remained independent. So given that hospitals and nursing homes in many of the rural communities are primary employers, we really have had huge impact on some of those communities. Are there some that struggle in spite of our presence? Absolutely. And they probably will. And health care there may not be sustained. But I think we've made a tremendous difference." Kathleen McGreevy and Russell McKnight, "Interview with **Carol DeSchepper**," February 9, 2010.

"How are people being treated? How are employees being treated? How do all of the health care workers in the hospital treat each other? So the board has major issues in oversight. They're not in there every day, but the board needs to be assured that those things are happening, that the hospital has a clear mission, a vision. That's planned out year by year in the strategic planning, and then that gives you also the measures that are happening as far as quality care. And, of course, now we have much more sophisticated measures for quality care which you can compare yourself on national figures and get a picture of: How are we doing as far as quality? The board has a responsibility to be monitoring those things, given to them by the CEO and the management team. Russell McKnight, "Interview with **Sister Mary Jaeger**," February 19, 2010.

"When I came to town in 1995, there were seven physicians in the McKennan network, and today we have about 350 physicians in about 80 locations. The Sisters' philosophy is that we meet people where they want to be met, and so we have never been out there actively pursuing physician practices; we've let them come to us, and I think a healthy part of the relationship is that they are the ones seeking out a partnership. There are lots of reasons why they might want to partner with us at a specific time. For some it's a computer system, for some it's recruitment. When we present to them, we always start with the mission and the vision. They need to know who we are. They need to know that we're comfortable with who we are and that there's some obligation on their part to follow our mission…. They want a strong local hospital; we want a strong local hospital. They want us to treat their employees right, and we want to treat their employees right. And so it's really the integrated approach that we believe in." Russell McKnight and Margaret Preston, "Interview with **David Flicek**," August 21, 2009.

"I've heard people say, 'Why can't we just go back to the good old days?' I think if we did, they'd be pretty selective because I don't think anybody wants to go back to a six- or eight-bed ward with no bathrooms. People might have liked the simplicity, but we always need to remember that we have opportunities in moving forward." Russell McKnight and Margaret Preston, "Interview with **LaVonne Gaspar**," August 28, 2009.

"There are many non-profit organizations around the country that found it easier to give things away than to nurture the resources they had. It was easy to make care available for free, but it was much harder to figure out a way to pay for it. We've always been able to balance the need for fiscal responsibility with our need to [fulfill] the charitable mission of the Sisters, and I think we've done a great job on that." Kathleen McGreevy, Russell McKnight and Margaret Preston, "Interview with **Fred Slunecka**," November 30, 2009.

"That early sense that I had of this being a calm, sort of sacred healing place is still there in many respects. Maybe it's there in my head more than anything. The nuns aren't a presence anymore. But I think the mission is still evident in this respect for patients, respect for families, respect for visitors. I think that's a really good thing." Russell McKnight, "Interview with **Fred Margot Nelson**," August, 2009.

Select Bibliography Original source materials

- *Aberdeen American News*
- *All of Us*
- *Argus Leader*
- *Bishop's Bulletin*, Sioux Falls Catholic Diocese
- Fifth Annual Report of the McKennan Hospital, 1916
- Minute Book of Trustees of the McKennan Hospital Fund
- Minute Book of Trustees of the McKennan Hospital
- *New York Times*
- *Orleans Republican*
- Presentation Nurse
- *Sioux City Journal*
- Voices and Ventures: A Newsletter for Friends of Sisters of the Presentation of the Blessed Virgin Mary

Secondary Sources

- Drudy, P.J., ed. *The Irish in America: Emigration, Assimilation and Impact* (Cambridge: Cambridge University Press, 1985).
- Fialka, John J. *Sisters: Catholic Sisters and the Making of America* (New York: St. Martin's Griffin, 2004).
- Fitzpatrick, M. Louise. *Prologue to Professionalism: A History of Nursing* (Maryland: Robert J. Brady, Co., 1983). Grauvogl, Ann. Committed to Care: A Century of Medical Education in South Dakota (Sioux Falls: Pine Hill Press, 2007).
- Harrington, Dolores. *A Woman's Will…A Sister's Way: The McKennan Hospital Story* (Sioux Falls: n.p., 1961).
- Karoleritz, Robert F. *With Faith, Hope and Tenacity: The First One Hundred Years of the Catholic Diocese of Sioux Falls: 1889-1989* (Mission Hill, SD: Dakota Homestead Publishers, 1989).
- Karolevitz, Robert F. A *Commitment to Care: The First 100 Years of Sacred Heart Hospital 1897-1997* (South Dakota: Pine Hill Press, Inc., 1997).
- Kingsbury, George W. *History of Dakota Territory, South Dakota; its History and its People* (ed.) George Martin Smith Vol. 5 (Chicago: S.J. Clarke Publishing, 1915).
- Kolata, Gina. *Flu: The Story of the Great Influenza Pandemic of 1918 and the Virus that Caused It* (New York: Firrar Straus and Giroux, 1999).
- McGreevy, Kathleen. *A Century of Care…A Journey of Faith: Avera Queen of Peace Hospital 1906-2006* (Mitchell: Avera Queen of Peace Health Services, 2006).
- Mooney, Margaret. *Doing What Needs to be Done: Sisters of the Presentation of the Blessed Virgin Mary, Fargo 1882-1997* (Fargo, ND Access Midwest, 1997).
- O'Farrell, Mary Pius. *Nano Nagle: Woman of the Gospel* (County Kildare: Presentation Generalate Monasterevin, 1996).
- Olson, Gary D. and Erik L. Olson. *Sioux Falls, South Dakota: A Pictorial History* (Virginia: Donning Company, 2003).
- Peterson, Susan Carol and Courtney Ann Vaughn-Roberson. *Women With Vision: The Presentation Sisters of South Dakota* (Urbana: University of Illinois Press, 1988).
- Preston, Margaret. *Charitable Words: Women, Philanthropy and the Language of Charity in Nineteenth-Century Dublin* (Connecticut: Praeger, 2004).
- Quinn, Sister Pauline. *Biographies of Mother Superiors*, (n.p., n.d.).
- Recker, Narcy. *An Institution of Organized Kindness* (Sioux Falls, Sioux Valley Hospital, 1996).
- Robinson, Ron. *Sioux Falls Construction: A Century of Building 1910-2010* (Sioux Falls: Solutions Media, 2010).
- Signor, Issac. *Landmarks of Orleans County* (Syracuse: D. Mason & Co., 1894).
- Stevens, Rosemary. *In Sickness and in Wealth: American Hospitals in the Twentieth Century* (Baltimore: John Hopkins University Press, 1999).
- Thomas, A. *Sketches of the Village of Albion* (Albion: Willsea & Brach, 1853).
- Steele, Volney. *Bleed, Blister and Purge: A History of Medicine on the American Frontier* (Montana: Mountain Press Publishing Co., 2005).
- Wall, Barbra. *Unlikely Entrepreneurs: Catholic Sisters and the Hospital Marketplace* (Columbus: Ohio State University Press, 2005).

Endnotes

1 "Sioux Falls Magnificent New Hospital under Construction," *Argus Leader*, January 28, 1911.

2 Dolores Harrington, *A Woman's Will…A Sister's Way: The McKennan Hospital Story* (Sioux Falls: n.p., 1961), p. 9.

3 "All…except $3,500, which was subscribed by the physicians and others of the city for part purchase of the hospital block, was borrowed—about $106,500." See "Explanation Called For President of McKennan Hospital Association Tells of Financial Condition," n.d., 1913 and "Publish the Will Trustees of McKennan Hospital Make Public the Donor's Will," n.d. Both articles most likely from the *Argus Leader*, located in Minute Book of Trustees of the McKennan Hospital Fund, Heritage Hall, Avera McKennan Hospital.

4 "Work on the Hospital," *Argus Leader*, June 21, 1911.

5 Kathleen McGreevy, "Interview with Mickey Billion," October 24, 2008. "Dr. Billion, Sister, Is Honored for 50 Year Medical Practice," *Argus Leader* n.d., 1951. According to Mrs. Billion, as young men, T.J. Billion and Thomas O'Gorman were roommates at St. Thomas Military Academy, a high school in St. Paul.

6 A note in the Trustee Minute Book on October 13, 1906, states that a motion was carried to accept an invitation from the "Sisters" of the hospital in Mitchell to attend the dedication services there. These "Sisters" were those of the Presentation Order who, in 1898, opened Notre Dame Academy in Mitchell and were already running St. Luke's Hospital which they established in Aberdeen in 1901. "Meeting October 13, 1906," Minute Book of Trustees of the McKennan Hospital Fund, Heritage Hall, Avera McKennan Hospital and Kathleen McGreevy, *A Century of Care…A Journey of Faith: Avera Queen of Peace Hospital 1906-2006* (Mitchell: Avera Queen of Peace Health Services, 2006), p. 13.

7 "Meeting, April 12, 1910," Minute Book of Trustees of the McKennan Hospital Fund, Heritage Hall, Avera McKennan Hospital and Dolores Harrington, *A Woman's Will*, p. 9.

8 "The McKennan Hospital Impressively Dedicated," *Argus Leader*, December 18, 1911.

9 "The M'Kennan Hospital Impressively Dedicated," *Argus Leader*, December 18, 1911.

10 "The M'Kennan Hospital Impressively Dedicated," *Argus Leader*, December 18, 1911.

11 "Golden Jubilee Program to End Thursday at McKennan," *Argus Leader*, June 21, 1961 and Harrington, *A Woman's Will*, p. 13-14.

12 Letter: Dr. G.I.W. Cottam to Sister Mary Coleman Coakley November 27, 1977—his misspelling.

13 "The M'Kennan Hospital Impressively Dedicated," *Argus Leader*, December 18, 1911. According to the *Argus Leader*, the hospital could accommodate 85 patients while Harrington notes 55. Harrington, *A Woman's Will*, p. 10.

14 Peter Temin, "An Economic History of American Hospitals," in Health Care in America H.E. French III ed. (California: Pacific Research Institute for Public Policy, 1988), p. 81.

15 Harrington, *A Woman's Will*, p. 20.

16 Sister Agatha was born Bridget Collins in County Cork Ireland in 1872; after serving at McKennan Hospital she was superior general of the Presentation Order from 1921 to 1927. Sr. Agatha Collins died in 1954.

17 "Hospital is Incorporated," *Argus Leader*, January 3, 1912 and Harrington, *A Woman's Will*, p. 94.

18 "Hospital 'Linen Shower' Great Success," *Argus Leader*, February 15, 1912.

19 "Mrs. M'Kennan Died this P.M.," *Argus Leader*, September 29, 1906. Edwin A. Sherman, 1844-1916, fought to ensure that McKennan's will was respected and that the 20 acres set aside for the park be honored. See "That M'Kennan House Matter," *Argus Leader*, November 30, 1906.

* There were two other sons: Sidney was born on February 4, 1835 and died March 4, 1861 and Wilbur was born March 21, 1843 and died August 16, 1844.

20 From "Galesburg Gales Reunion October 4, 1986—revised August 21, 1993," in archives of First Congregationalist Church, Fern L. Chamberlain author—kind thanks to Ms. Janice Nims and First Congregational Church for supplying information on McKennan, her brother Artemus and A.E. Sherman.

21 "Death of Dr. McKennan," *Orleans Republican* August 27, 1879. Guild and McKennan had three children. Issac Signor, Landmarks of Orleans County (Syracuse: D. Mason & Co., 1894), pp. 140, 191, 263, 610 and 648. See also A. Thomas, *Sketches of the Village of Albion* (Albion: Willsea & Brach, 1853), p. 20 and Orleans County Directory 1969, p. 127.

22 Gary D. Olson and Erik L. Olson, *Sioux Falls, South Dakota: A Pictorial History* (Virginia: Donning Company, 2003), p. 21 and Ann Grauvogl, "Helen McKennan Her Legacy is a City Park, A Hospital," *Argus Leader* May 1, 1983.

23 http://www.siouxfalls.org/Information/history/park_history/McKennan. aspx; David Richardson and Sioux Falls Planning and Building Services Department, "McKennan Park Historic District," (n.p., n.d.) and Larry Weires "A Trilogy of Sioux Falls Park History," *Pioneer Pathfinder* Vol. 35, No. 1 (January, 2009), p. 3.

24 Mrs. George E. Cox, *First Congregational Church: A Congregation of the United Church of Christ Centennial 1872-1972* (n.p., 1971), located in Caille room Sioux Falls Main Library.

25 "Mrs. M'Kennan Died this P.M.," *Argus Leader*, September 29, 1906. Apparently, the gift was made despite objections from her family. See Grauvogl, "Helen McKennan Her Legacy."

26 "A Good Woman Gone," *Argus Leader*, October 2, 1906.

27 "Hospital for Sioux Falls," *Argus Leader*, October 2, 1906, pp. 1-2. Helen's brother, Artemus, was the recipient of some of her estate.

28 "Need A Hospital," *Argus Leader*, August 20, 1906. Dr. Sebaikin-Ross has his own interesting history. See Robert F. Karoleritz, *With Faith, Hope and Tenacity: The First One Hundred Years of the Catholic Diocese of Sioux Falls: 1889-1989* (Mission Hill, SD: Dakota Homestead Publishers, 1989), p. 58.

* Mallanney's name can be found with a variety of spellings. The *Argus Leader*, spelled his name Mallaney and the Sioux Falls directory spelled it Malanny. Harrington's spelling of Mallanney will be used. Harrington, *A Woman's Will*.

29 George W. Kingsbury, *History of Dakota Territory, South Dakota; its History and its People* (ed.) George Martin Smith Vol. 5 (Chicago: S.J. Clarke Publishing, 1915), pp. 1054-1056. The author would like to thank Kevin Gansz curator of education for the Old Courthouse Museum for his assistance in locating this information.

30 Olson, *Sioux Falls, South Dakota*, p. 25.

31 Stanley K. Schultz and Clay McShane, "To Engineer the Metropolis: Sewers, Sanitation, and City Planning in Late-Nineteenth-Century America," *The Journal of American History*, Vol. 65, No. 2 (Sept. 1978), p. 407

32 Harrington, *A Woman's Will*, p 71.

33 Volney Steele, *Bleed, Blister and Purge: A History of Medicine on the American Frontier* (Montana: Mountain Press Publishing Co., 2005), pp. 167-9.

34 See Peter Temin, "An Economic History of American Hospitals," pp. 80-81.

35 "Sioux Falls Hospital," *Argus Leader*, August 30, 1894.

36 In addition to the physicians, the hospital's new staff also included two trained nurses from the Lutheran Deaconess Order. See Narcy Recker, *An Institution of Organized Kindness* (Sioux Falls, Sioux Valley Hospital, 1996), pp. 2-5; Olson, *Sioux Falls, South Dakota*, p. 77.

37 Harrington, *A Woman's Will*, p. 90.

38 Recker, *An Institution of Organized Kindness*, pp. 7-8 and 14-17 and "Sioux Valley Hospital Now Being Operated in Full Force," *Argus Leader*, July, 30, 1930.

39 Olson, *Sioux Falls, South Dakota*, pp. 121 and 146; "Patient Comfort Must be Guarded," *Argus Leader* September 20, 1950; Harrington, *A Woman's Will*, p. 91 and http://www.cchs.org/about/history.

40 Into the 21st century, Catholic hospitals remain the "largest single group of the nation's not-for-profit hospitals…." Barbra Wall, *Unlikely Entrepreneurs: Catholic Sisters and the Hospital Marketplace* (Columbus: Ohio State University Press, 2005), pp. 3, 22; 33-34.

41 Patrick J. Blessing "Irish emigration to the United States, 1800-1920: An Overview," *The Irish in America: Emigration, Assimilation and Impacted*. P.J. Drudy (Cambridge: Cambridge University Press, 1985), p. 21.

42 Mary Pius O'Farrell, *Nano Nagle: Woman of the Gospel* (County Kildare: Presentation Generalate Monasterevin, 1996), pp. 61-62.

43 Presentation ties to their Irish roots were strong. For example, in Aberdeen, up until the 1950s, only native-born Irish women were elected as the convent's mother superior.

44 McCabe Papers Ref. No 346 1-4 Shelf 331 II (1880). Papers located in Dublin Diocesan Archives.

45 Camillus M. Galvin, *From Acorn to Oak: A Study of Presentation Foundations 1775-1968* (Fargo, N.D.: Presentation Sisters, 1969), p. 63 and Sister Mary Margaret Mooney, *Doing What Needs to be Done: Sisters of the Presentation of the Blessed Virgin Mary, Fargo 1882-1997* (Fargo, ND Access Midwest, 1997), p. 23.

46 Susan Carol Peterson and Courtney Ann Vaughn-Roberson, *Women With Vision: The Presentation Sisters of South Dakota* (Urbana: University of Illinois Press, 1988), p. 65.

47 Butler, Mother Joseph, Annals 1880-1915 Box 10.3, Folder 2.

48 Peterson and Vaughn-Roberson, *Women With Vision*, pp. 164-195. By 1911, in addition to St. Luke's, the order was running St. Joseph's in Mitchell, SD (1906), Holy Rosary in Miles City, Montana (1910) and McKennan Hospital (1911) in Sioux Falls.

49 Harrington, *A Woman's Will*, p. 21 and Fifth Annual Report of The McKennan Hospital (1916), Presentation Archives 102.5 Box 13 F3, pp. 3-4. By this time the population of Sioux Falls was over 20,000.

50 "Archduke and Duchess of Hohenberg Assassinated," *Argus Leader*, June 29, 1914.

51 "U.S. Enters World War; German Ships Seized," *Argus Leader*, April 6, 1917.

52 "Sammies Have No Epidemics," *Argus Leader*, March 7, 1918.

53 David M. Morens, Jeffery K. Taubenberger, and Anthony S. Fauci, "Predominant Role of Bacterial Pneumonia as a Cause of Death in Pandemic Influenza: Implications for the Pandemic Influenza Preparedness," *Journal of Infectious Diseases* 198 (1 October 2008), pp. 1-2.

54 "No Danger of Epidemic of Spanish Grip," *Argus Leader*, September 18, 1918.

55 "Spanish Grip is Spreading Rapidly East," *Argus Leader*, September 25, 1918; "Stamping out Spanish Grip War Measure," *Argus Leader*, September 26, 1918, p. 1; "Cancel Draft Calls Because of Epidemics," *Argus Leader*, September 27, 1918 and "Grip in Army Better; Spreads with Civilians," *Argus Leader*, October 3, 1918.

56 "Sioux City Schools Closed," *Argus Leader*, October 8, 1918, p. 1; "Close all Public Places But Schools," *Argus Leader*, October 12, 1918. See also Rhonda Keen-Payne, "We Must Have Nurses: Spanish Influenza in American 1918-1919," *Nursing History Review* 8 (2000), pp. 143, 149-151, 154.

57 Gina Kolata, *Flu: The Story of the Great Influenza Pandemic of 1918 and the Virus that Caused It* (New York: Firrar Straus and Giroux, 1999), pp. ix-x, 80 and G.R. "Experiences during the Influenza Epidemic," *The American Journal of Nursing* Vol. 19, No. 3 (Dec., 1918), pp. 203-205.

58 "Flu Worst Enemy of State During 1918; Takes Toll of 1,847," *Argus Leader*, May 8, 1919.

59 Harrington, *A Woman's Will*, p. 23 and Karoleritz, *With Faith, Hope and Tenacity*, p. 173; Harrington does not state the number of pneumonia cases at McKennan. Renke also talks about the flu taking a toll on Sioux Valley Hospital where "corridors, offices and even the parlor were used to house the patients." Renke, *An Institution of Organized Kindness*, p. 10.

60 Anonymous Typed Manuscript (1911-1918), McKennan Hospital Scrapbook # 3, Presentation Archives.

61 Harrington, *A Woman's Will*, p. 26.

62 "McKennan Hospital Cancels $25,000 Outstanding Bonds," *Argus Leader*, n.d.

63 "Addition to M'Kennan Hospital, to be Built this summer, Will Make it One of Finest in West," *Argus Leader*, June 18, 1918 and "Extension to McKennan Hospital is Rapidly Nearing Completion," *Argus Leader* November 9, 1918. According to Harrington the cost came to $180,056.15.

64 Stevens, *In Sickness and in Wealth*, p. 111.

65 Harrington, *A Woman's Will*, p. 26.

66 Stevens, *In Sickness and in Wealth*, p. 115.

67 Sister Pauline Quinn, "Mother Raphael McCarthy 1932-1946," Biographies of Mother Superiors, Presentation Archives.

68 Harrington, *A Woman's Will*, pp. 30-31. The debt was fully paid off in 1947. Harrington, *A Woman's Will*, p. 39.

69 Kathleen McGreevy, ed. "Diploma Graduates of 1927…Share Memories, Laughter," *All of Us* Vol.14, 3 (May/June 1992), pp. 4-5.

70 Peterson and Vaughn-Roberson, *Women with Vision*, p. 102.

71 Mother Raphael McCarthy to Mr. W. A. Rawlings, Vice President, Massachusetts Mutual Life Insurance Company, July 1, 1934; Presentation Archives Mother Raphael 10.6 Box 1 F 5.

72 Peter Temin, "An Economic History of American Hospitals," p. 86.

73 Mother Raphael McCarthy to Mr. W. A. Rawlings, July 1, 1934.

74 Mother Raphael McCarthy to Mr. William C. Olson, Cashier, Massachusetts Mutual Life Insurance Company, April 23, 1936, Presentation Archives, McCarthy, Raphael 10. 6 Box 1 F 5.

75 Mother Raphael McCarthy to Mr. W. A. Rawlings, Vice President, Massachusetts Mutual Life Insurance Company, July 7, 1936; Presentation Archives, McCarthy, Raphael 10. 6 Box 1 F 5.

76 Mr. Neil J. Gleason, President Neil J. Gleason & Co to Mother Raphael McCarthy, December 8, 1942; Presentation Archives, McCarthy, Raphael 10.6 Box 1, F 3.

77 Mr. Neil J. Gleason, President Neil J. Gleason & Co to Mother Raphael McCarthy, December 8 and 15, 1942, my emphasis. Presentation Archives, McCarthy, Raphael 10.6 Box 1 F 3; my emphasis. $17,810,887.59 using the nominal GDP per capita; see www.measuringworth.com/.

78 Mr. Neil J. Gleason, President Neil J. Gleason & Co to Mother Raphael McCarthy, March 20, 1944; Presentation Archives, McCarthy, Raphael 10.6 Box 1 F 4. Thanks to Mr. Rick Lundberg for clarification of accounting terminology.

79 Mr. Neil J. Gleason, President Neil J. Gleason & Co to Mother Raphael McCarthy, June 20, 1945 10.6 Box 1 F 3.

80 This information is based on a 1946 tally by Peterson and Vaughn-Roberson, Women with Vision p. 108

81 "Congressional Record Proceedings and Debates of the 86th Congress, Second Session," Vol. 106, No. 30, Washington, D.C., Thursday, August 11, 1969.

82 McCarthy had corneal scarring and cataracts. After the surgery, McCarthy expressed joy in seeing clouds in the sky, the host during mass and being able to read her missal and office book. Mother Raphael McCarthy 10.6 Box 1, Folder 1 Presentation Archives.

83 Sister Pauline Quinn, "Biographies of Mother Superiors: Mother Raphael McCarthy 1932-1946," p. 7. Oral Interview with Sisters Colman Coakley, Annrita Johnson, SaBina Joyce, Suzanne Cotter, Bernadette Farrell and Mary Thomas May 13, 2008.

* Nodlaig is Irish for Christmas.

84 Julie Sanchez, "Forty Years of Caring," *All of Us* Vol. 14, No. 6 (November/December 1992), p. 2. Irish born Sister Borgia Fitzgerald worked in McKennan's business office. She died on August 14, 1980.

85 Kathleen McGreevy, "McKennan Hospital Expanding to Serve a Growing Community," *All of Us* Vol. 14, No. 4 (July/August 1992), pp. 4-5.

86 Voices and Ventures A Newsletter for Friends of Sisters of the Presentation of the Blessed Virgin Mary Vol. 4, No. 2 (Spring 1996).

87 Kathleen McGreevy, "Interview with Paul Connelly," December 17, 2007.

88 Don Bierle, general counsel of Avera Health died on October 10, 2002. See Kathleen McGreevy, ed., "In Memory: Don Bierle," *All of Us* Vol. 24, 1 (Jan./Feb./Mar., 2002), p. 10.

89 Kathleen McGreevy, "Businesswoman and Missionary" South Dakota Hall of Fame (Fall, 1997). Dr. Patrick McGreevy nominated Sister Colman Coakley.

90 Kathleen McGreevy and Margaret Preston "Interview with Sister Colman Coakley", September 30, 2008 and January 30, 2009; Ann Grauvogl, "Missionary Spirit: Sister Vows to Care for Sick as Chairwoman of the Board," *Argus Leader* April 29, 1984; "Sister Colman—A Woman with a Mission," *All of Us* n.d. and Kathleen McGreevy and Margaret Preston, "Interview with John Hughes," May 27, 2009.

91 "Jubilee," Voices & Ventures: A Newsletter for Friends of the Sisters of the Presentation of the Blessed Virgin Mary, Aberdeen, S.D. Vol. 18, 1 (June, 2010), p. 15 and "Six to celebrate 60 years, one to mark 70 years with Aberdeen convent," *Argus Leader* July 4, 2010.

* Crimean War (1853-1856); U.S. Civil War (1861-1865).

92 Women philanthropists had an important role in the changes to nursing. See Regina Markell Morantz, "Making Women Modern: Middle Class Women and Health Reform in 19th Century America," *Journal of Social*

History Vol. 10, 4 (1977), pp. 490-507; Susan Armeny, "Organized Nurses, Women Philanthropists, and the Intellectual Bases for Cooperation Among Women, 1898-1920," *Nursing History New Perspectives, New Possibilities* ed. Ellen Condlifee Lagemann (New York: Teachers College Press, 1983), p. 33; Patricia O'Brien D'Antonio, "The Legacy of Domesticity Nursing in Early Nineteenth-Century America," *Nursing History Review* 1 (1993), pp. 229-46 and Margaret Preston, *Charitable Words: Women, Philanthropy and the Language of Charity in Nineteenth-Century Dublin* (Connecticut: Praeger, 2004).

93   Steele, *Bleed, Blister and Purge*, p. 245.

94   Anonymous Typed Manuscript (1911-1918), McKennan Hospital Scrapbook, # 3, Presentation Archives.

95   Kathleen McGreevy, "Interview with Dorcas Baldwin," January 17 and 20, 2006.

96   Letter to Directors of Hospitals from Thomas Parran, U.S. Surgeon General, July 20, 1943. Cadet Nursing Program Correspondence, Presentation Archives.

97   "Federal Security Agency U.S. Public Health Service Division of Nurse Education" Form 40---July 1943, Cadet Nursing Program Correspondence, Presentation Archives and "Uniforms and Insignia of U.S. Cadet Nurse Corps Chosen," *Aberdeen American News* September, n.d., 1943.

98   St. Luke's became the hospital's "headquarters" due to its proximity to Northern State Teacher's College whose faculty, early on, provided science courses. Susan Peterson and Amy K. Reiger, "'They Needed Nurses at Home' The Cadet Nurse Corps in South and North Dakota," *South Dakota History* Vol. 23, No. 2 (1993), pp. 124-125.

99   Peterson and Reiger, "They Needed Nurses at Home," p. 124; Peterson and Vaughn-Roberson, *Women With Vision*, p. 208; Harrington, *A Woman's Will*, pp. 35-37; "S.F. Nurses Observe Anniversary," *Argus Leader*, November 14, 1948 and "Four Nursing Schools to Be Combined Here," *Aberdeen American News* (nd, 1945).

100   *The Presentation Nurse* Vol. 1, No. 4 (February, 1943), p. 1.

101   M. Louise Fitzpatrick, *Prologue to Professionalism: A History of Nursing* (Maryland: Robert J. Brady, Co., 1983), p. 51.

102   In 1945, with the help of a federal grant of over $67,000, McKennan restored the Bishop's residence and renamed it St. Mary's Hall. "Work on $100,000 Nurses' Home at McKennan Hospital Completed," *Argus Leader* April, n.d., 1945.

103   "Departments at McKennan Gain Beds," *Argus Leader* May 28, 1961; "Historic Building Yields to Progress," Bishop's Bulletin, Sioux Falls Catholic Diocese, November-December 1972, p. 3; "Landmark Razed for Expansion," *Argus Leader* January 19, 1973, p. 8 and Kathleen McGreevy and Margaret Preston, "Interview with Sister Colman Coakley," September 30, 2008. Brady served as Bishop from 1939-1946.

104   Kathleen McGreevy, "Interview with Sister Colman Coakley," February 23, 2006.

105   For discussion of nursing's struggles during the late 19th and early 20th centuries see Susan M. Reverby, *Ordered to Care: The Dilemma of American Nursing 1850-1945* (Cambridge: Cambridge University Press, 1987).

106   Peterson and Vaughn-Roberson, *Women with Vision* pp. 147-48 and http://www.presentation.edu/aboutPC.htm.

107   Harrington, *A Woman's Will*, p. 49-50; "Presentation School of Nursing has Enrolled," *Argus Leader* July 22, 1958 and "Nursing School Ready," *Argus Leader*, n.d., 1951. The school admitted the first male students in 1951. "Golden Jubilee Program to End Thursday at McKennan," *Argus Leader* June 21, 1961.

108   "McKennan Will Close Nurse School," *Argus Leader* July 25, 1965.

*   McKennan Hospital became Avera McKennan Hospital on September 9, 1998. See discussion below.

109   Steve Young, "Nurses Celebrate 50th Anniversary," *Argus Leader*, July 30, 1995.

110   Joyce Terveen, "Nurses Seek Cure for Image," *Argus Leader* April 30, 1989 and Joyce Terveen, "Schedule Helps Mom Split Time Between Work, Family," *Argus Leader* April 30, 1989. See also, "Nursing's Come A Long Way, Baby," *Argus Leader* April, nd, 1991.

111   Kathleen McGreevy, ed., "Celebrating Nursing in its Many Different Forms," *All of Us* Vol. 23, 3 (July/Aug./Sept., 2001), pp. 10-12 and "Avera McKennan Gains National Recognition for Nursing Excellence," Avera McKennan News Room January 21, 2010.

112   Donna Farris, "Excellence in Nursing," Avera McKennan White Paper May 2008.

113   Kathleen McGreevy and Margaret Preston, "Interview with Judy Blauwet," December 2, 2008.

*   Helicopter or fixed-wing emergency transport.

114   Donna Farris, "Excellence in Nursing," May 2008.

115   "Gilbert Cottam, 75, Former S.F. Doctor, Dies at Pierre," *Argus Leader* March 4, 1949.

116   Harrington, *A Woman's Will*, p. 76. Gilbert Cottam died in 1949.

117   "Dr. Cottam Recalls Surgery 'First' in South Dakota" *Argus Leader* n.d. 1969. In 1977, Dr. Cottam wrote to Sister Colman of his recollections about the procedure and stated that the tumor was inoperable but he had enlarged the skull in order to relieve the pressure, and the patient lived on for quite some time. Letter: Dr. G.I.W. Cottam to Sister Mary Coleman Coakley, November 27, 1977—his misspelling of her name.

118   Scientists had experimented with electric shock to the hearts of animals since the 19th century. It was first tried on a human in 1947 and conducted only with the chest cavity open until the early 1950s.

119   Kathleen McGreevy, "Interview with Vernon Ronald "V.R." Nelson," May 26, 2009 and Vern Loen, "'Heart Shocker' May Save Lives Here," *Argus Leader* June 20, 1954. Dr. Geoffrey Cottam died at McKennan Hospital on October 14, 1984. "School of Medicine Loses Dear Friend" Internal McKennan Newsletter, n.d. 1984, located in Scrapbook #58, Presentation Archives.

120   Ralph Green, "Shock Usage, Heart Message, Save Life of Hartford Man," *Argus Leader* n.d., 1958.

121   "Augustana Donates Defibrillator," *Argus Leader*, n.d. and "Dr Vernon Ronald Nelson," *South Dakota Magazine* (Sept/Oct 2008), p. 83. Nelson was inducted into the South Dakota Hall of Fame in 2008 for his many inventions including the electronic control system for the Zip Feed Mill and the first electronic football scoreboard at Augustana College. An early version of Nelson's shocker is held in the Sioux Empire Medical Museum located at Sanford Hospital.

122   "Dr. S.A. Donahoe, 78, Dies Suddenly in SF," *Argus Leader* May 3, 1966. S.A. Donahoe was born on November 8, 1887 in Sioux Falls. In a 1973 letter from Will Donahoe to Sister Colman, Donahoe recollected that he and his cousin, Dr. S.A. Donahoe, delivered ice to the vicinity of the hospital while attending medical school. Letter to Sister M. Coleman, Administrator from W.E. Donahoe, February 19, 1973—his misspelling of her name. Presentation Archives 102.5 Box 1, F 1.

123   In 1940, eight years after Bishop Bernard Mahoney asked Mother Raphael McCarthy to take over the operation of the diocesan children's home that had been destroyed by fire in 1932, the Presentation Children's Home of Sioux Falls opened and would, over the years, house up to 90 children of all denominations. Peterson and Vaughn-Roberson, *Women with Vision* pp. 104-105. However, as federal demands and increased understanding of the psychology of childrearing became more complicated, "…by 1965 the Presentations decided that they had ventured out of their area of professional specialty…" and closed the home.

124   Honora Mary Burns was born in Rowena, SD in 1892 and entered the novitiate in 1914. The first Mother Superior born in the United States, she succeeded Mother Raphael McCarthy in 1946. She died in 1966. Peterson and Vaughn-Roberson, *Women with Vision*, pp. 109-111.

125   "Distinguished Service Award Honors Dr. Will E. Donahoe," *Argus Leader*, n.d.; "Dr. Will Donahoe Receives 1960 Frank Owens Award," *Argus Leader* May 23, 1960; Letter: Dr. Will E. Donahoe, M.D. to Mother M. Viator, Superior McKennan Hospital, June 19, 1961, Presentation Archives 102.5 Box 13 F 2; "Citizen of the Week," *Argus Leader* September 13, 1964; "Dr. Donahue heads McKennan Staff," *Sioux Falls Suburban News* January 26, 1967; "Dr. Will E. Donahoe, Age 85, Reminisces; is Still Practicing," *Argus Leader* May 7, 1972 and Dr. Donahoe, "Longtime Physician in Sioux Falls, Dies at Age 89," *Argus Leader* December 22, 1975.

126   "New Clinic to Cost $60,000," *Argus Leader* March 10, 1919.

127   "Dr. Guy Van Demark Retiring After 42 Years of Practice," *Argus Leader* n.d. 1949 and "Dr. Guy Van Demark Dies at 84; Funeral Tuesday," *Argus Leader* November 9, 1963.

*   "New Pregnancy Test Used $8 Frogs Housed in McKennan Lab," *Argus Leader* April 10, 1948. Sadly, the story turns tragic. It seems that the Xenopus laevis, which made its way into obstetrician's office throughout the world, is the source of a deadly fungus that is contributing to the mass death of large

numbers of the frogs throughout the world. See Elizabeth Kolbert, "The Sixth Extinction?" *The New Yorker* May 25, 2009, pp. 53-56. Thanks to Russell McKnight pointing out this article.

128 Olson, *Sioux Falls, South Dakota*, p. 137.

129 Kathleen McGreevy, ed., "Setting the PACE…" *All of Us* Vol. 14, No. 6 (November/December 1992), p. 9; Kathleen McGreevy, ed., "PHS Joins Nation's Largest Purchasing Alliance," *All of Us* Vol., 18, 2 (April/May 1996), pp. 11-12; Kathleen A. McGreevy, "A History of Avera Health," unpublished paper (September 2001) and http://www.avera.org/avera/pace/index.aspx.

130 *The Presentation Nurse*, Vol. I, No. 1 (November, 1943), p. 1.

131 For example, while in 1873 there were 178 hospitals in the United States, by 1909 there were 4,357; then between 1909 and 1946 hospital numbers increased by 44 percent. Paul A. Brinker and Burley Walker "The Hill-Burton Act: 1948-1954," *The Review of Economics and Statistics* Vol. 44, 2 (May, 1962), pp. 208-212.

132 Ralph W. Green, "Golden Jubilee Anniversary Edition," *Argus Leader* June 18, 1961, p. 2; "Public Inspection Set for Sunday," *Argus Leader* n.d. 1943 and *The Presentation Nurse*, Vol. II, No. 4 (February, 1944), p. 1.

133 Harrington, *A Woman's Will*, p. 38 and *The Presentation Nurse* Vol. IV, No. 3 (June, 1946), p. 9.

134 *The Presentation Nurse*, 4 (February 1944), p. 2. Note that this number includes bassinets. In 1931 McKennan also built a wing onto the hospital that included a chapel and classrooms. Harrington, *A Woman's Will*, p. 32.

135 Russell McKnight, "Interview with Margot Nelson" August, 2009 and Russell McKnight and Margaret Preston, "Interview with LaVonne Gaspar," August, 2009.

136 Russell McKnight and Margaret Preston, "Interview with Kay Brink," August, 2009.

137 Kathleen McGreevy, "Interview with Sister Colman Coakley," February 23, 2006.

138 Stevens, *In Sickness and in Wealth*, p. 262.

139 "Harkison General Chairman of McKennan Fund Campaign," *Argus Leader* n.d., 1955.

140 "McKennan Hospital," *Argus Leader*, n.d. 1953.

141 "Harkison General Chairman of McKennan Fund Campaign," *Argus Leader* n.d., 1955.

142 "S.F. Physicians Seek to Raise $100,000 of McKennan Fund; Seven Pledge $23,500 Total," *Argus Leader* n.d. and "Doctors Over Quota for McKennan Fund," *Argus Leader* n.d.

143 "McKennan Expansion Fund is Explained to Businessmen," *Argus Leader* n.d. 1955?. According to the *Argus Leader*, from 1942-1952 the number of children born at the hospital increased by 130% from 672 in 1942 to 1,433 in 1952. "McKennan Hospital," *Argus Leader*, n.d., 1953.

144 "McKennan fund at $401,699 As Employees Give $13,562," *Argus Leader*, February 20, 1954.

145 Peterson and Vaughn-Roberson, *Women With Vision*, p. 178; "Colleges and Hospitals Get Huge Grants Half Billion in Ford Foundation Funds Sets U.S. Precedent," *Sioux City Journal* December 19, 1955; "McKennan Hospital $350,000 Fund Drive Planned," *Argus Leader* n.d., 1955; "McKennan Expansion Fund is Explained to Businessmen," *Argus Leader* n.d. 1955?; "S.D. Hospitals Get Ford Grants," *Argus Leader* December 13, 1955; "Contracts for Building of McKennan Addition Awarded," *Argus Leader* June 19, 1955 and "16 S.D. Hospitals Getting Ford Aid," *Argus Leader* April 8, 1956.

146 Paul A. Brinker and Burley Walker, "The Hill-Burton Act: 1948-1954," The Review of Economics and Statistics Vol. 44, No. 2 (May, 1962), pp. 208-211; Stevens, *In Sickness and in Wealth*, p. 227 and Bess Furman, "Hospital-Aid Plan Has 347 Projects," *New York Times* July 2, 1948.

147 Harrington, *A Woman's Will*, p. 47; "Plans Changed for McKennan Construction," *Argus Leader* August 19, 1954; "$250,000 Is Granted for 2 Hospitals," *Argus Leader* n.d. 1955; "Expansion Program at McKennan Hospital to Begin About July 1," *Argus Leader* n.d., 1956; "McKennan's New Look," *Argus Leader* October 20, 1957 and "Many See New McKennan Wing," *Argus Leader* October 27, 1957.

148 See, "More Federal Participation In Health, Medical Fields Forecast," *Argus Leader* October 26, 1960.

149 "McKennan Hospital Advisory Board Formed," *Argus Leader* January 27, 1956. In 1960 McKennan built a new surgical unit of 22 beds. See "Facts about McKennan Hospital for 1960," *McKennan News* n.d., Presentation

Archives 102.5 McKennan Hospital Box 1 F1; Ralph Green, "New Unit Adds 22 Surgical Beds at McKennan Hospital," *Argus Leader* January 3, 1960 and "McKennan Hospital to Add $175,000 Two-Floor Wing," *Argus Leader* April 19, 1964.

150 Kathleen McGreevy, "Interview with Sister Colman Coakley," February 23, 2006.

151 "Roosevelt's Own Creed Set Forth," *New York Times* August 6, 1912; Hugh O'Connor, "New Deal Pushes Medical Care Plan," *New York Times* October 27, 1938; "Million Hold Hospital Insurance," *New York Times* February 13, 1938; "Health Insurance Covers Half of US," *New York Times* September 13, 1951; Edward A. Marciniak, "Public Health Insurance in the United States," *American Catholic Sociological Review* Vol. 8, 3 (October 1947), pp. 188-192 and Melissa A. Thomasson, "From Sickness to Health: The Twentieth-Century Development of U.S. Health Insurance," *Explorations in Economic Theory* 39 (2002), p. 233.

152 John D. Morris, "President Signs Medicare Bill; Praises Truman," *New York Times* July 30, 1965.

153 Stevens, *In Sickness and in Wealth*, pp. 284; 286-7.

154 John J. Fialka, *Sisters: Catholic Sisters and the Making of America* (New York: St. Martin's Griffin, 2004), p. 217.

155 Helen Rose Ebaugh, Jon Lorence and Janet Saltzman Chafetz, "The Growth and Decline of the Population of Catholic Sisters Cross-Nationally, 1960-1990: A Case of Secularization as Social Structural Change," *Journal for the Scientific Study of Religion* 35, 2 (1996), pp. 174-175; Peter Steinfels, *A People Adrift: The Crisis of the Roman Catholic Church in America* (New York: Simon & Schuster), pp. 278-279; Fialka, *Sisters*, p. 200 and Laurie Goodstein, "U.S. Sisters Facing Vatican Scrutiny," *New York Times* July 2, 2009.

156 Fialka, *Sisters*, p. 301.

157 Kathleen McGreevy, ed., "Mary Clare Julson," *All of Us* Vol. 14, No. 4 (July/August 1992), p. 6.

158 Kathleen McGreevy, "Interview with Jim Ward," January 10, 2006.

159 Kathleen McGreevy, "Interview with Jim Ward." Jim Ward retired in 1995.

160 The first Chief Operating Officers of the hospital were given the title Superior and Administrator. Over the years, the title changed.

161 Kathleen McGreevy, "Interview with Henry Morris," January 15, 2007.

162 Stevens, *In Sickness and in Wealth*, pp. 293-94.

163 Slunecka became Avera's chief operating officer on September 1, 2010. See "Fred Slunecka Named to New COO Position at Avera Health," *Argus Leader*, August 26, 2010.

164 Kathleen McGreevy, Russell McKnight and Margaret Preston, "Interview with Fred Slunecka," July 30, 2009. It is interesting to note that private rooms were not a new asset for McKennan; when the hospital opened in 1911 it offered 30 private rooms—half of which had private baths.

165 "Sioux Falls Hospitals Face Bed Shortage," *Argus Leader* November 18, 1980 and "Overcrowded McKennan Wants an Addition," *Argus Leader* January 10, 1981.

166 "Local Hospitals Expand to Meet Area Medical Needs," *Argus Leader* March, 3, 1981.

167 Stevens, *In Sickness and in Wealth*, pp. 323-324 and Robert Pear, "Reagan Asking Wide Changes in Nation's Health Insurance System," *New York Times* March 1, 1983.

168 Kathleen McGreevy and Russell McKnight, "Interview with Carol DeSchepper," February 9, 2010.

169 Stevens, *In Sickness and in Wealth*, pp. 297; 300.

170 Ann Grauvogl "Hospitals Vie for Patients," *Argus Leader* September 12, 1985.

171 Ann Grauvogl "Hospital Boom Goes Bust with Layoffs" *Argus Leader* September 2, 1984 and "Medical Care Bumper Crop Planted by Post-War Aid," *Argus Leader* September 2, 1984.

172 Ann Grauvogl, "Hospitals face Dilemma: McKennan has Too Few Patients, Sioux Valley Has Too Many" and "American Hospitals are in Financial Trouble, Health Economist Says," *Argus Leader* March 20, 1983.

173 Lisa Ryan, "McKennan Administrator Quits," *Argus Leader* December 2, 1983.

174 Ann Grauvogl, "City Hospitals Wage Ongoing Battle for Patients," *Argus Leader* January 1, 1984.

175 Kathleen McGreevy, "Interview with Dr. Richard Hosen," August 15, 2006. McKennan also experienced two very tragic events. In November of 1982,

a woman was abducted from the McKennan parking ramp and murdered. In January of 1986, a patient was given the wrong blood type which resulted in her death. These terrible events weighed heavily on the hospital and it sought to learn from them by, among other things, improving security of parking areas and changing the system for handling blood. Lisa Ryan, "Escorts in Demand at McKennan Hospital," *Argus Leader* November 15, 1982; Brenda Wade, "McKennan Absolved from Slaying," *Argus Leader* March 7, 1986; Jim Rasmussen, "Family Sues Hospital Over Blood Mistake," *Argus Leader* August 9, 1986 and Jim Rasmussen, "Fatal Mistake Changes Hospital Policy," *Argus Leader* March 2, 1986.

176 Mark V. Pauly, "A Primer on Competition in Medical Markets," ed. H.e. Frech III Health Care in America: The Political Economy of Hospitals and Health Insurance (San Francisco: Pacific Research Institute for Public Policy, 1988), pp. 98-99; Grauvogl, "Hospitals face Dilemma" and Ann Grauvogl, "Sioux Falls: Progress on the Plains," Corporate Report March 1982, p. 94, Presentation Archives 102.5 Box 13, F1.

177 Kevin Lollar, "Hospitals at Odds Over Heart Program," *Argus Leader* August 18, 1986 and Julie Bolding, "McKennan gets OK for Heart Program," *Argus Leader* December 27, 1986. See also Kathy McGreevy and Margaret Preston, "Interview with Jon Soderholm," July 16 and 20, 2009.

178 McGreevy, "McKennan Hospital" p. 5.

179 Joyce Terveen, "Partners to Open $40M Heart Hospital," *Argus Leader* March 10, 1999 and Kathleen McGreevy and Margaret Preston, "Interview with Mr. John Colman Hughes," May 27, 2009.

180 Kevin Dobbs "Stakes Now Higher in S.D. Heart Battle," *Argus Leader* March 11, 2001; Kevin Dobbs, "Compact Size Yields Efficiency, Officials Say," *Argus Leader* March 11, 2001; Kevin Dobbs "Why Doctors Want to Own a Hospital," *Argus Leader* March 13, 2001 and Kevin Dobbs "Heart Doctors Triggered Health Care Shift," *Argus Leader* December 28, 2003.

181 Joyce Terveen "Heart Hospital Top Project in City History," *Argus Leader* October 2, 1999.

182 Kathy McGreevy and Margaret Preston, "Interview with Jon Soderholm," July 16, 2009.

183 Megan Myers, "Hospitals Battling for Hearts," *Argus Leader* November 5, 2007 and Megan Myers, "Ruling Frees Heart Hospital," *Argus Leader* August 14, 2006.

* Sanford Hospital, formerly Sioux Valley Hospital, changed its name in 2006. See discussion below.

184 Jon Walker, "Sanford Hospital Raises Heart Debate," *Argus Leader*, April 19, 2010.

185 Fred Slunecka, "E-mail to Avera McKennan Sioux Falls and Regional Employees," August 30, 2010.

186 Ann Grauvogl, *Committed to Care: A Century of Medical Education in South Dakota* (Sioux Falls: Pine Hill Press, 2007), pp. 101-105.

187 Grauvogl, *Committed to Care*, pp. 109 and 116.

188 Kathleen McGreevy, "Interview with Henry Morris," January 15, 2007 and Grauvogl, *Committed to Care*, pp. 107 and 117.

189 See "Affiliation Agreement: The University of South Dakota/McKennan Hospital," 102.5 Box 1 F 4, Presentation Archives.

190 Grauvogl, *Committed to Care*, pp. 124, 127; 131 and 135.

191 McGreevy, "Interview with Henry Morris." See also, Kathleen McGreevy, "Interview with Dr. Richard Hosen" August 15, 2006 and Kathleen McGreevy, "Interview with Loren Amundson" June 23, 2008.

192 Grauvogl, *Committed to Care*, p. 148

193 "Avera McKennan Announces Addition to Name," Avera McKennan Press Release, March 31, 2000 and Joyce Terveen "The Hospital Name Game," *Argus Leader* May 14, 2000.

194 Grauvogl, Committed to Care, p. 157 and Kenyon Gleason, "Avera Offers 14 New Annual Scholarships for Medical Students at the U," Avera McKennan News Room October 6, 2006.

195 Megan Myers, "Avera Gift Might be SDSU Record," *Argus Leader* November 7, 2007 and Jamie Ziemer "Hospital Systems Spreading Wealth," *Argus Leader* December 5, 2007.

196 Russel McKnight, "Interview with Kimberlee and Jennifer McKay," May 20, 2010.

197 The first participants, all graduates of American medical schools, were Drs. Rose Faithe, David Ritzenthaler, James Hockenberry and Neil Elkjer.

198 The residency's first director was Dr. Lloyd Sweeney; the associate director was Dr. Loren Amundson. McKennan is also host to several "flexible" interns each year.

199 Kathleen McGreevy, "Interview with Dr. Al Hartman," December 17, 2009 and Kathleen McGreevy, "Interview with Dr. Loren Amundson," June 23, 2008.

200 To implement technological advances in patient care, hospitals now needed more specialized workers. At various times and as needs evolved, McKennan Hospital offered a School of Radiology Technology, a School of Medical Technology, a School of Anesthesia and a School of Respiratory Therapy. The hospital continues to serve as a clinical practice site for students who learn these and other health-related disciplines in colleges and technical schools.

201 McGreevy and Preston, "Interview with Jon Soderholm."

202 "Joining the Fight Against Cancer," *Argus Leader* May 11, 1991.

203 Rob Swenson, "Surgical Center, Cancer Institute Details Coming," *Argus Leader* April 16, 2008; Rob Swenson, "Avera Envisions World-Class Cancer Care," *Argus Leader* April 30, 2008 and Megan Myers, "We Need to Be Ahead of the Community's Needs," *Argus Leader* May 8, 2008.

204 "Life's Transformation Through Grace and Technology," Avera McKennan Foundation, 2009.

205 See Ron Robinson, *Sioux Falls Construction: A Century of Building 1910-2010* (Sioux Falls: Solutions Media, 2010), pp. 67-73.

206 Rob Swenson, "Avera Envisions World-Class Cancer Care"; Donna Farris "World-Class Cancer Care: New Avera Cancer Institute Offers Comprehensive Care, Right Here at Home," Avera McKennan White Paper August, 2008; News from the Avera McKennan Foundation (Winter, 2009), p. 2 and "Life's Transformation through Grace and Technology," Avera Cancer Institute, 2009.

207 Avera McKennan has commissioned "an exquisite collection of commissioned art to bring comfort and inspire hope" and these pieces are throughout the building as well as its external grounds. Russel McKnight and Margaret Preston, "Interview with Richard Molseed," August 21, 2009.

208 Kathleen McGreevy and Margaret Preston, "Interview with Patricia "Patty" Peters, MD," June 19, 2009.

209 Megan Myers "Big Plans for Avera Cancer Center," *Argus Leader* April 22, 2008 and Rob Swenson, "Avera Envisions World-Class Cancer Care."

210 Kathy McGreevy, Russell McKnight and Margaret Preston, "Interview with Fred Slunecka," July 30, 2009. Avera McKennan Hospital also offers a sculpture walk to enhance the hospital's aesthetics. See "Indoor Sculpture Walk at Avera Good for Patients, Visitors," *Argus Leader* June 24, 2010.

211 Megan Myers, "Avera: Surgery Center Crucial," *Argus Leader* March 30, 2008.

212 Donna Farris, "Avera Surgery Center: Combining Medical Expertise and the Latest Technology with 5-Star Service," Avera McKennan White Paper, July 2010.

213 Farris, "Avera Surgery Center," p. 2. See also, Jon Walter, "$93 Million Avera Cancer Institute Unveils Surgery Center," *Argus Leader* July 6, 2010.

214 "Avera McKennan Granted $2,492,032 for First-of-its Kind Cancer Treatment for the Region from the Leona M. and Harry B. Helmsley Charitable Trust" Avera Health News Release February 23, 2010.

215 Joyce Terveen "Transplant Unit Planned," *Argus Leader* July 8, 1992; Grauvogl, Committed to Care, pp. 149; 151; Todd Nelson, "State's First Kidney Transplant Brotherly Act," *Argus Leader* July 10, 1993; "First Kidney Transplant at McKennan," All of Us Vol. 15, 5 (August/September 1993), p. 4 and Grauvogl, Committed to Care, p. 151.

216 Jamie Ziemer, "Sioux Valley, McKennan Say Demand is Strong," *Argus Leader* November 1, 2006.

217 See Kathleen McGreevy, ed., "Avera McKennan Transplant Institute Earns Approval For Pancreas, as well as Kidney and Bone Marrow Transplants," All of Us Vol. 26, 1 (Jan/Feb/Mar 2004), p. 9.

218 Jamie Ziemer, "Avera Prepares to Add Livers to Transplant Program," *Argus Leader* October 15, 2008; Jamie Ziemer, "Sioux Valley, McKennan Say Demand is Strong"; "Avera Transplant Institute Performs 500th Solid Organ Transplant" Avera McKennan News Room and Donna Farris, "Transplant Program Grows in Strength," Avera McKennan White Paper January, 2009.

219 See John T. Porter, "Becoming a System," All of Us Vol., 19, 1 (February/March 1997), p. 3.

220 Marsha Gold, "The Changing US Health Care System: Challenges for Responsible Public Policy," The Milbank Quarterly Vol., 77, 1 (1999), p.7 ; See also Jamie Ziemer "Independent Doctors Weight Freedom vs. Systems' Support," *Argus Leader* January 16, 2008.

221 "Central Plains Clinic, LTD," *Eyes on You Magazine* (1992) and Dr. Loren Amundson, "Historical Marker Text" Etc. for Her (April, 2006), p. 46. The historical marker dedicated to the Donahoe clinic sits at 9th Street and First Avenue in Sioux Falls.

222 Todd Nelson "Local Clinic Moves East," *Argus Leader* March 20, 1992.

223 Russell McKnight and Margaret Preston, "Interview with Fred Slunecka," July 30, 2009.

224 Kevin Dobbs, "Hospital Competition Extends to Central Plains," *Argus Leader* March 11, 2001.

225 Kathleen McGreevy, "Interview with Dr. Pat McGreevy," July 11, 2007.

226 Russell McKnight and Margaret Preston, "Interview with David Flicek," August 2009.

227 For example see, Kathleen McGreevy, ed., "Iowa Hospital Managed by McKennan," *All of Us* Vol. 16, 5 (October/November 1994), p. 3.

228 McKnight and Preston, "Interview with David Flicek."

229 Robert F. Karolevitz, *A Commitment to Care: The First 100 Years of Sacred Heart Hospital 1897-1997* (South Dakota: Pine Hill Press, Inc., 1997), pp. 19-21 and http://www.yanktonbenedictines.org.

230 Kathleen McGreevy, "A History of Avera Health," unpublished paper (August, 2001) updated by Clare Willrodt, June, 2009, p. 8.

231 Kathleen McGreevy, ed., "Benedictine, Presentation Health Systems Link Services," *All of Us* Vol. 18, 3 (June/July 1996), p. 3; 5.

232 Kathleen McGreevy, "A History of Avera Health," p. 10.

233 John Porter, "Becoming 'Avera Health'" *All of Us* Vol. 20, 2 (April/May, 1998), p. 3.

234 Robert Voglewede, "An Interview Regarding Co-sponsorship" (Summer, 2001).

235 Kathleen McGreevy, ed., "Avera Health: A New Name for Presentation Health System," *All of Us* Vol. 20, 5 (April/May 1998), p. 5. McKennan did not officially change its name until September 9, 1998. See Kathleen McGreevy, ed., "Celebration," *All of Us* Vol. 20, 5 (October/November, 1998), pp. 5-11.

236 Joyce Terveen, "Presentation to be renamed Avera Health," *Argus Leader* March 12, 1998.

237 Russ McKnight and Margaret Preston, "Interview with Sister Mary Thomas," August, 2009; see also Joyce Terveen, "McKennan gets a Name Change," *Argus Leader* September 9, 1998.

238 McKnight and Preston, "Interview with David Flicek."

239 Kathleen McGreevy and Margaret Preston, "Interview with Becky Severson and Norma Steinocker," November 6, 2008.

240 Jamie Ziemer, "McKennan Projects to Add Rooms, Increase Privacy" *Argus Leader* August 16, 2006 and Jamie Ziemer, "Avera Expects More Patients in Revamped ER" *Argus Leader* December 5, 2007.

241 Lean manufacturing or lean production, often simply, "Lean," is a production practice that considers the expenditure of resources for any goal other than the creation of value for the end customer to be wasteful, and thus a target for elimination. Basically, lean is centered on preserving value with less work. http://en.wikipedia.org

242 Donna Farris, "Leading the Way with LEAN" Avera McKennan White Paper September, 2007.

243 "eEmergency Goes Live October 15," *All of Us* Vol. 31, No. 4 (Fall, 2009), p. 1 and Steve Young, "Long-Distance Medicine," *Argus Leader* January 8, 2010.

244 Steve Young, "Long-Distance Medicine,"; Jamie Ziemer, "Gift to Kick-Start Telehealth," *Argus Leader* April 29, 2009 and Margaret Preston, "Interview with Amanda Bell," June 18, 2010.

245 Chul-Young Roh, "Telemedicine: What it is, Where it Came From, and Where it Will Go," Comparative Technology Transfer and Society Vol., 6 No., 1 (April, 2008), pp. 37-40 and Nancy Brown, "A Brief History of Telemedicine" Telemedicine Information Exchange (May 30, 1995), p. 2 http://tie.telemed.org/articles/article.asp?path=articles&article=tmhistory_nb_tie95.xml

246 Clare Willroot, ed., "Gifts to Avera Will Revolutionize Rural Health, "*All of Us* Vo. 31, 2 (Spring, 2009), p. 1.

247 Kathleen McGreevy, ed., "Telemedicine: It's Here, or Almost Here, and Some Say it Will Transform Rural America," *All of Us*, Vol. 16, 1 (February/ March 1994), pp. 1-3.

248 Clare Vanbrandwijk, ed., *All of Us* Vol. 26, 4 (Fall, 2004), p. 1.

249 "Telemedicine Saves Lives, Money, Avera Study Finds," *Argus Leader* April 15, 2009 and "Avera Study Shows Positive Impact of Remote Intensivist Care through eICU" Avera McKennan News Room, April 9, 2009.

250 Donna Farris, "Bringing Quality Care, Close to Home: Advancing Technology Fosters Growth of Avera Telehealth," Avera McKennan White Paper December, 2007; "Avera Study Shows Positive Impact of Remote Intensivist Care through eICU" Avera McKennan News Room, April 9, 2009 and "Avera Receives Telehealth Award" *Argus Leader* June 11, 2009.

251 Ralph Green, "Memorial Established at McKennan to Pay Tribute to Sister Matthew," *Argus Leader* n.d.1954.

252 Kathleen McGreevy, "Interview with Dr. Russell Orr," July 19, 2006.

253 Green, "Memorial Established at McKennan to Pay Tribute to Sister Matthew."

254 Kathleen McGreevy, "Interview with Eleanor "Mickey" Billion," October 24, 2008.

255 Green, "Memorial Established at McKennan to Pay Tribute to Sister Matthew," and Harrington, *A Woman's Will*, p. 43.

256 Anonymous Typed Manuscript (1911-1918), McKennan Hospital Scrapbook, 3, Presentation Archives.

257 Green, "Golden Jubilee Anniversary Edition," *Argus Leader* June 18, 1961, p. 2 and Margaret Preston, "Interview with Albena Reinke," October 28, 2008. See also, Harris Simons, "Like White House, McKennan Nursery Installs Rockers," *Argus Leader* July 2, 1961.

258 "College Nursing Program Includes Individualized Mother-Baby Care," *Argus Leader*, n.d., 1970.

259 Kathleen McGreevy and Margaret Preston, "Interview with Becky Severson and Norma Steinocker," November 6, 2008.

260 Todd Nelson, "McKennan Addition to Serve Women, Kids," *Argus Leader* February 28, 1992 and Kathleen McGreevy, ed., "McKennan Women's and Children's Centers" *All of Us* Vol. 15, 5 (August/September 1993), p. 3. Ultimately it appears that LDRP rooms, while nice for the parents, are expensive and inefficient in hospitals the size of McKennan. As demand increased, the hospital needed the delivery rooms free and once again women are moved from delivery room to a separate hospital room. Margaret Preston, "E-mail correspondence with Becky Severson," Wednesday June 23, 2010.

261 Donna Farris "Caring for Kids: Avera Children's offers top-quality, comprehensive Pediatric Services" Avera McKennan White Paper, March 2009.

262 "Psychiatric Ward Opens at McKennan Hospital Monday," *Argus Leader*, September 14, 1958.

263 "Treatment for Mental 'Illness' is Mental 'Health'," *Argus Leader* May 9, 1976.

264 "Program Hopes to Fill Void in Adolescent Psychiatric Care," *Argus Leader* September 11, 1977 and "McKennan Shifts Focus," *Argus Leader* April 17, 1978.

265 Jamie Tanata, "Avera's New Center Surpasses Trends," *Argus Leader* April 5, 2006. In 2004, Avera McKennan purchased Sioux Valley Hospital's inpatient behavioral health facility.

266 Kevin Dobbs, "Avera to Build Mental Hospital," *Argus Leader* April 24, 2004. See also Jamie Tanata, "Avera's New Center Surpasses Trends," *Argus Leader* April 5, 2006; Megan Myers "A Stigma, Made Largely of Fear and Misunderstanding Lingers Over Mental Health Issues Today," *Argus Leader* March 19, 2006 and "Hospital Plans Welcome," *Argus Leader* May 3, 2004.

267 Kelly Hildebrandt, "Hospital to Offer Serenity, Security," *Argus Leader* June 12, 2005; Jamie Tanata, "Avera's New Center Surpasses Trends," *Argus Leader* April 5, 2006 and Donna Farris, "A Regional Leader: Growth of Avera Behavioral Health Services Exceeds Expectations" Avera McKennan White Paper, March, 2008.

268 Farris, "A Regional Leader"; Tanata, "Avera's New Center Surpasses Trends," *Argus Leader* April 5, 2006 and Jay Kirschenmann, "Original Art a Prominent Priority in New Health Center," *Argus Leader* April 2, 2006.

269 Megan Myers, "National Organization Applauds Quality of Avera McKennan Services," *Argus Leader* July 29, 2009.

270 Pat Mack, "Musical Duet: Avera Project Helps Children Develop and Research Flourish," South Dakota M.D. (Spring/Summer, 2010), p. 20.

271 Donna Farris, "Advancing the Science of Behavioral Health," Avera McKennan White Paper, July 2008.

272 Farris, "Advancing the Science of Behavioral Health."

273 Terry Wooster, "New Preschool Project Could Rekindle Dispute," *Argus Leader*, August 10, 2008; "Avera Reaching Kids Strengthening Family

Wellness," Avera McKennan Foundation (Winter, 2009) and "Recital Showcases Talents for Family and Friends," Avera McKennan Foundation (Summer, 2009).

274   Mack, "Musical Duet: Avera Project Helps Children Develop and Research Flourish," p. 20.

275   "Hospital for Sioux Falls," Argus Leader October 2, 1906, pp. 1-2.

276   Stephen R. Connor, "Development of Hospice and Palliative Care in the United States," Journal of Death and Dying Vol. 56, No., 1 (2007-2008), pp. 91-93 and Vincent W. Franco, "The Hospice: Humane Care for the Dying," Journal of Religion and Health Vol 24, No. 1 (Spring, 1985), p. 80.

277   "McKennan Opens 4-Bed In-house Hospice," All of Us (March, 1987?), n.p.

278   Kathleen McGreevy, ed., "PHS Unites Hospital, Long-Term Care Services" All of Us Vol. 16, 5 (October/November 1994), p. 1.

279   Megan Myers, "$1M Gift Boosts Hospice Residence," Argus Leader October 22, 2005 and Megan Myers, "The Dougherty Hospice House," Argus Leader July 26, 2006.

280   Megan Myers, "Avera McKennan to Build Hospice," Argus Leader October 21, 2005. Megan Myers, "Compassionate Care to the End," Argus Leader December 1, 2007; Kenyon Gleason, "New Dougherty Hospice House Enhances End of Life Care," Avera McKennan News Room November 30, 2007.

281   Jamie Ziemer, "Avera to Ease Hospice Need with New Facility," Argus Leader September 20, 2006.

282   William Dougherty, who was born April 6, 1932, was inducted into the South Dakota Hall of Fame in 2009; he died on July 3, 2010. David Kranz, "Exiting the Lobby," Argus Leader May 6, 2009 and Jonathan Ellis, "Dougherty, Democratic Force and Ally of Kennedys, Dies at 78," Argus Leader July 4, 2010.

283   Kathleen McGreevy and Margaret Preston, "Interview with William "Bill" Dougherty," April 3, 2008.

284   This was not a surprising direction for McKennan to go in as, other than the federal government, Catholic health care is the greatest source of free health care throughout the United States. Fialka, Sisters, pp. 301-2.

285   Gary Umland, "The Bridge," South Dakota Academy of Physicians Assistants Vol. 6, Issue 2 (May, 1996), p. 6.

286   Joyce Terveen, "McKennan Expanding Clinic," Argus Leader April 24, 2000.

287   Margaret Preston and Robin Prunty, "Interview with Joanne Hindbjorgan and Dr. James Barker," May 21, 2009.

288   Randy Hascall, "Uninsured Patients Flock to Free Clinic," Argus Leader August 10, 1993. See also Matt Cecil, "McKennan Planning Free Clinic," Argus Leader July 18, 1992; Rich Naser, "Follow up: Free Clinic Filling Up Fast," Health Care Community News, n.d and Joyce Terveen, "Lack of Insurance Driving Working Poor to Free Clinics," Argus Leader October 7, 1997.

289   Kathleen McGreevy and Margaret Preston, "Interview with Jeremiah Murphy" May 27, 2008 and September 9, 2008 and Russ McKnight and Margaret Preston, "Interview with Sister Mary Thomas," August 21, 2009.

290   Ralph Green, "A Minister's Views of on the Hospital," Argus Leader June 18, 1961, p. 3.

291   "The M'Kennan Hospital Impressively Dedicated," Argus Leader December 18, 1911.

292   http://www.acpe.edu/WhoWeAreHistory.html

293   "Six Complete Pastoral Care Course…" All of Us, (n.d. 1974), Scrapbook #16, Presentation Archives.

294   Gail Richardson, "Clergy Learn to Deal with the Dying," Argus Leader n.d.

295   Fr. Lawrence Murtagh died on December 2, 2005 at the age of 78. See "ACPE and North Central Region Lose a True Elder," ACPE News of the North Central Region Vol. XXXVIII, No. 4 (December, 1995), p. 1.

296   Kathleen McGreevy, ed., "Clinical Pastoral Education: Learning Through Daily Caring," All of Us Vol. 13, No. 4 (September/October 1991), p. 2 and Margaret Preston, "Interview with Peter Holland and Steven Corum," July 28, 2010.

297   Kathleen McGreevy and Margaret Preston, "Interview with Clara Johnson," July 15, 2009.

298   The original Nano Nagle Inn opened in 1995 as a guest house for families of bone marrow transplant patients. Kathleen McGreevy, ed. "Nano Nagle Inn Opens Near McKennan," All of Us December 1995, p. 11.

299   Wolf also sculpted "To Be Well" which sits in front of the Avera Health building in Sioux Falls. See Kathy McGreevy, ed., "New Sculpture," All of Us Vol. 26, 3 (July/August/September, 2004), pp. 6-7.

300   Darwin Wolf "Carlitos the Brave" Artist Statement 2008; "Walsh Family Village" Avera McKennan Foundation, (2007-2008 Annual Report) and http://www.loscaboschildren.org/Index.aspx?p=1; see also, Mark Stuertz, "Foundation of Hope," American Way February 1, 2010, pp. 22-25.

301   Harrington, A Woman's Will, p. 17. See David H. Smith, "McKennan's Long Service to Humanity Chronicled," Argus Leader August 5, 1962 and "Herb Bechtold's Round Robin," Argus Leader September 5, 1962.

302   Kathleen McGreevy, "Interview with Dr. Russell Orr," July 19, 2006.

303   Russel McKnight and Margaret Preston, "Interview with Linda Olson," August 21, 2009.

304   Benda Wade, "Seniors Decide Meal Beats Eating Alone," Argus Leader December n.d., 1986? and Todd Nelson, "Sioux Falls Celebrates Holiday in Varied Ways," Argus Leader December 26, 1988.

305   Kathleen McGreevy, ed., "Christmas Day Dinner," All of Us Vol. 13, 6 (Christmas, 1991), p. 2. and Kathleen McGreevy, ed., "Christmas Feasts," All of Us Vol. 15, 7 (Christmas, 1993), p. 1.

306   McKnight and Preston, "Interview with Fred Slunecka,"; Russ McKnight, "Avera McKennan Annual Report Video," 2009 and Clare Willrodt, ed. "Avera Donates Ambulance to Crow Creek Sioux Tribe," All of Us Vol. 30, 4 (Fall, 2008), p. 3.

307   Kathleen McGreevy and Margaret Preston, "Interview with Mr. John Colman Hughes," May 27, 2009. See also, Bob Voglewede, "The Sisters," All of Us Vol. 19, 3 (June/July, 1997), p. 13.

308   Harrington, A Woman's Will, p. 32.

309   In 1938, the Auxiliary initiated a student loan fund in order to assist the school of nursing. Harrington, A Woman's Will, pp. 32-33 and Anonymous, Typescript (1945) located in scrapbook # 14 Presentation Archives. See also Letter to Auxiliary from Cecilia Donweiler, R.N., n.d. 1942 scrapbook #14 Presentation Archives.

310   Dean Belbas, "Charity Ball Adds to McKennan Assets," Argus Leader n.d., 1950; "McKennan Isolette One of First in Area," Argus Leader March 3, 1953; "St Mary's Nurses Student Lounge," Argus Leader, n.d., 1955 and "Auxiliary to buy Hospital Bed," Argus Leader April 17, 1960. See also, Kathleen McGreevy, "Interview with Sister Colman Coakley," February 23, 2006.

311   "'April in Paris' gaiety for Charity Ball," Argus Leader Sunday April 15, 1962 and "Nearly $10,000 Donated by Auxiliary to Hospital," Argus Leader May 15, 1962. See also, letter from Peggy Muchow and Madeline Haering of Occupational Therapy November 12, 1962 Scrapbook #14 Presentation Archives and "McKennan Ball to Feature New Setting, Art, 2 Bands," Argus Leader April 2, 1978.

312   "Golden Jubilee Program to End Thursday at McKennan," Argus Leader n.d., 1961; Barbara Hoffbeck, "Students Donate Time, Talent to Hospitals," Argus Leader August 12, 1962 and "Candy Stripers, B'Nai B'rith Unit Get Youth Awards," Argus Leader October 20, 1962.

313   "Betty Elkjer, 89, Helped Start Hospital Volunteerism," Argus Leader March 16, 2001. Elkjer, born in 1911 in Hancock Minn., moved to Sioux Falls with her husband in 1949 where she began her more than 20-year career at McKennan. See also Grace Nelson, "Pink Ladies Lend Cheerful Aid," Argus Leader May 7, 1961 and "Candy-Stripers are Teen-age Volunteers at Hospital," Argus Leader September 17, 1961.

314   Ann Grauvogl "Hospital Volunteers," Argus Leader November 28, 1984.

315   Robert Voglewede, "The Sisters," All of Us Vol. 19, 3 (June/July 1997), p. 13 and Russel McKnight, "Interview with Jennifer and Kimberlee McKay," May 20, 2010.

Margaret Preston is an Associate Professor in the History Department at Augustana College. The author of Charitable Words: Women, Philanthropy and the Language of Charity in Nineteenth-Century Dublin (Praeger, 2004), she received her Ph.D. in history from Boston College in 1999.

1911-1925 McKennan Hospital's First Board of Directors

Colonel Thomas H. Brown, President

Mother Joseph Butler

Dr. Edwin L. Perkins

Mr. John Mallanney

Bishop Thomas O'Gorman

Oscar A. Brown
(joined in 1922 with death of Thomas H. Brown)

Most Rev. Bernard J. Mahoney
(joined in 1923 with death of Bishop Thomas O'Gorman)

Harold E. Judge
(joined in 1923 after the death of John Mallanney)

1925-present Board members

(Year indicates when service began on the board)

Mother Cecelia O'Sullivan	1925
Mother Agatha Collins	1925
Rev. Mother Raphael McCarthy	1925
Rev. Mother Viator Burns	1926
Mother Aloysius Chriswell	1925, 1927
Mother Joseph Butler	1925, 1928
Sister Francis Holland	1925, 1928
Sister Ursula Conroy	1939
Mother Bonaventure Hoffman	1939, 1955
Sister Monica Parkinson	1940
Sister Borgia Fitzgerald	1940
Mother Cornelia Swanton	1946
Sister Evarista Reddy	1952
Sister Bernadette Farrell	1952, 1963
Mother Leona Kallas	1952
Sister Camillus Shealy	1955
Sister Leonard Fitzgerald	1955
Sister Bernard Quinn	1955, 1968
Sister Richard Caron	1956
Sister Rita Janish	1957
Rev. Mother Carmelita McCullough	1958
Sister Colman Coakley	1958
Sister Vincent Fuller	1961
Sister Alma Staudenraus	1963
Rev. Mother Myron Martin	1964
Sister Conception Hamilton	1964

Sister Corita Dickinson	1964
Sister Marian Peter	1964
Sister Gonzaga Jeanette Silvis	1966, 1974
Sister Judith O'Brien	1966
Sister Mary Ellen Kaskie	1967
Sister Katherine Scholtz	1967
Sister Antonia Dunn	1970
Sister Irene Talbott	1970
Louis Hurwitz	1970
Steve Everist	1970
J.O. Harrington	1970
Sister Bonnie Jean Wek	1971, 1989
Sister Lynn Marie Welbig	1971
Mr. William Heimerman	1971
B. Scott Reardon II	1971
Sister Mary Jaeger	1972
Sister Marian Peter	1972
Dr. Charles Balcer	1973
L.R. Hurwitz	1973
Dempster Christenson	1973
Sister Miriam Therese Bowar	1975
Sister Phyllis Marie Calmus	1975
John Hulse	1975
Sister Nivard Farrell	1976
Dr. F.C. Kohlmeyer	1976
Sister Annrita Johnson	1977
Sister Aileen Huettl	1977
Sister Mary Schneider	1977
Sister Dominic Stoltz	1977
Charles Kearns	1977
David Billion	1977
Jeremiah Murphy	1977
Dan Wiedemeyer	1977
C.P. Moore	1977
Sister Sheila Schnell	1978
Lowell C. Hansen II	1978
Robert Atkins	1978
H. Lauren Lewis	1978
Sister Donna Brown	1979
Sister Elizabeth Remily	1979
Wayne H. Peters	1979
Sister Lucille Welbig	1980
Sister Virginia Calmus	1981

Board members (cont.)

Dr. S.M. Brzica	1982
William Dougherty	1982
Vance Goldammer	1982
Sister Rita Janish	1983
Richard McCrossen	1983
Gerald Sweetman	1983
Rudy J. Hoffman	1984
John Hughes	1984
Ed Gerloff	1984
Sister Marie Celeste Sabers	1985
Dr. J.P. Ingvoldstad	1985
Dr. Dennis L. Johnson	1985
Don Bierle	1985
Dr. Pat McGreevy	1986
Dr. G.D. Loos	1986
Karen Dunham	1986
Gary Junso	1986
Sister Ann Patrick Gannon	1987
Paul Connelly	1988
Steve Kirby	1988
Bruce Odson	1989
Dr. Lowell J. Hyland	1989
Ron Williamson	1989
Dr. Michael W. Pekas	1990
Dr. J.H. Hoskins	1990
James Smiley	1990
Dr. P.A. Peters	1992
Susan Scott	1992
Brad Grossenburg	1993
J. Tom Nelson	1993
Linda Laskowski	1993
Sister Virginia McCall	1994
Jack Marshman	1995
Rob Oliver	1995
Mike Brzica	1996
Dr. Leonard Gutnik	1996
Dr. Donald Wingert	1996
Sister Mary Jane Gaspar	1997
Robert Winkels	1998
Dr. John Sall	1998
Sister Joan Reichelt	1998

Scott Petersen	1998
Sister Kathryn Easley	1999
Sister Mary Denis Collins	1999
Dan Murphy	1999
Steve Crim	1999
Fred Slunecka	2000
Jerry Klein	2000
Mary Pat Sweetman	2000
Steve Billion, MD	2000
Walter Carlson, MD	2000
Jim McMahon	2001
Steve Pate	2001
Rob Everist	2002
John Griffin, MD	2002
Kim Pederson, MD	2002
Tom Dempster	2004
Jack Keers	2004
Steven Olson, MD	2004
Gayle Reardon, DDS	2004
Brad Thaemert, MD	2004
Farid Kutayli, MD	2006
Dave Rozenboom	2007
Fred Thurman	2007
Sister Candyce Chrystal	2008
Cathy Clark	2009
Michael Bender	2009
Mitchell Johnson, DO	2009
Sister Janice Klein	2009
Gene Jones Jr.	2009
David Fleck	2010
James Wiederrich	2010
David Chicoine, PhD	2011
Cindy Walsh	2011
William Rossing, MD	2011

1911-present Board Chairpersons

Col. Thomas H. Brown	1911
Oscar A. Brown	1922
Mother Cecelia Sullivan	1926
Mother Agatha Collins	1935
Rev. Mother Raphael McCarthy	1940

Board Chairpersons (cont.)

Rev. Mother Viator Burns 1946

Rev. Mother Carmelita McCullough 1958

Rev. Mother Myron Martin 1964

Sister Colman Coakley 1970

John Hughes 1989

Paul Connelly 1992

Jeremiah Murphy 1996

Pat McGreevy, MD 1999

Jack Marshman 2000

Rob Oliver 2002

Steve Crim 2004

Mary Pat Sweetman 2006

Rob Everist 2008

Tom Dempster 2010

Administrators

Mother Agatha Collins, *Administrator* 1911-1921

Sister Cecelia Sullivan, *Administrator* 1921-22; 1923-27

Sister Ligouri Lloyd, *Administrator* 1922-1923

Mother Raphael McCarthy, *Administrator* 1927-1932

Mother Agatha Collins, *Administrator* 1932-1940

Sister Monica Porkinson, *Administrator* 1940-1946

Mother Cornelia Swanton, *Administrator* 1946-1952

Sister Evarista Reddy, *Administrator* 1952-1954

Mother Bonaventure Hoffman, *Administrator* 1955-1964

Sister Corita Dickinson 1964-1970

Henry J. Morris 1970-1984

Roger Paavola 1984-1989

Fred Slunecka 1989-2010

Dr. David Kapaska 2010-present

Medical staff presidents/Chiefs of Staff

T.J. Billion Sr., MD 1919-1924

J.B. Gregg, Sr., MD 1925-1928

M.A. Stern, MD 1929-1930

R.G. Stevens, MD 1931-1932

R.J. Mullen, MD 1933-1934

P.R. Billingsley, MD 1935-1936

R. Reagan, MD 1937-1938

N.J. Nessa, MD 1939-1940

G.A. Stevens, MD 1941-1942

Gilbert Cottam, MD 1943

W.E. Donahoe, MD 1944

O.C. Ericksen, MD 1945

S.A. Donahoe, MD 1946-1947

C.J. McDonald, MD 1948

G.I. Cottam, MD 1949

L.J. Pankow, MD 1950-1951

W.F. Sercl, MD 1952

W.A. Arneson, MD 1953

R.E. Van Demark, MD 1954

M.S. Grove, MD 1955

M.W. Eggers, MD 1956

R.R. Donahoe, MD 1957

T.J. Billion Jr., MD 1958

J.V. McGreevy, MD 1959

C.S. Larson, MD 1960-1961

T.R. Anderson, MD 1970-1972

M.R. Ferrell, MD 1972-1974

Russell Orr, MD 1974-1976

S.M. Brzica, MD 1976-1978

J.J. Billion, MD 1978-1980

V.V. Volin, MD 1980-1982

N.J. Elkjer, MD 1982-1984

G.D. Loos, MD 1984-1986

Dennis L. Johnson, MD 1986-1988

P.S. McGreevy, MD 1988-1990

L.J. Hyland, MD 1999-1992

P.A. Peters, MD 1992-1994

A.E. Hartmann, MD 1994-1996

W.O. Carlson, MD 1996-1998

John Sall, MD 1998-2000

Donald Wingert, MD 2000-2003

Kim Pederson, MD 2003-2005

Farid Kutayli, MD 2005-2009

David Strand, MD 2009-Present

Sisters who have worked and volunteered at Avera McKennan 1911-2010

Aberdeen
Presentation Sisters

Sr. Agatha Collins

Sr. Rose McCormick

Sr. Magdalene Murphy

Sr. Xavier Treacy

Sr. Berchmans O'Brien

Sr. Elizabeth Prior

Sr. Justinian Wiseman

Sr. Ursula Conroy

Sr. Philomena Brennan

Sr. Assumpta Casey

Sr. De Chantal Duffy

Sr. Ligouri Lloyd

Sr. Xavier Shealy

M. Viator Burns

Sr. Cecelia O'Sullivan

Sr. Leonard Fitzgerald

Sr. Frances Therese Joyce

Sr. Cornelia Swanton

Sr. Berchmans Foley

M. Raphael McCarthy

Sr. Theophane Pennell

Sr. William Cody

Sr. Luke Drendel

Sr. Camillus Shealy

Sr. Alberta Mohaw

Sr. Patrick O'Reilly

Sr. Esther Blotz

Sr. Florence Hunegar

Sr. Jane Frances Lamm

Sr. Juliana Doohen

Sr. James Kelly

Sr. Joseph Freimuth

Sr. Matthew Brady

Sr. Bonaventure Hoffman

Sr. Denise Dauwen

Sr. Monica Parkinson

Sr. Borgia Fitzgerald

Sr. Gertrude Nemmers

Sr. Irene Talbot

Sr. Eileen Zeig

Sr. David Dorn

Sr. Evarista Reddy

Sr. Ambrose Muldoon

Sr. Scholastica Lemmer

Sr. Fidelis Ducan

Sr. Timothy Ryan

Sr. Regina Cotter

Sr. Marietta Rourke

Sr. Dominic Stoltz

Sr. Eugenia Hedigan

Sr. Eucharia Kelly

Sr. Claudia McNamara

Sr. Donald Burke

Sr. Mary Daley

Sr. Richard Caron

Sr. Esther Healy

Sr. Bernadette Farrell

Sr. Colman Coakley

Sr. Leona Kallas

Sr. Lucy Callaghan

Sr. Petrina McKee

Sr. Andre Schaub

Sr. Bernard Quinn

Sr. Rita Janish

Sr. Corita Dickinson

Sr. Mary Deis

Sr. Mary Aileen Huettl

Sr. Marian Peter

Sr. Theodora Paul

Sr. Madeleine Hohn

Sr. Antonia Dunn

Sr. Joanna Kellen

Sr. Roberta Rehbein

Sr. Alma Staudenraus

Sr. Martin Schuster

Sr. Vernon Huntimer

Sr. Edith Brandner

Sr. Geraldine Staudenraus

Sr. Noel Kuntz

Sr. Vincent Fuller

Sr. Michael Ann Mullaney

Sr. Janice Mengenhauser

Sr. Francine O'Connor

Sr. JoAnn Sturzl

Sr. Conception Doyle

Sr. Rosaria O'Callaghan

Sr. Charles Dresch

Sr. Celine Kelly

Sr. Gabriella Crowley

Sr. Janette Gaspar

Sr. De Pazzi Zimprich

Sr. Elizabeth Ann Marker

Sr. Irene Abeln

Sr. Nivard Farrell

Sr. Joan Maher

Sr. Mary Jaeger

Sr. David Ann Self

Sr. Joan Hillard

Sr. Kathleen Zimmer

Sr. Maria Gunn

Sr. Mary Burkey

Sr. Mary Ellen Kaskie

Sr. Miriam Zieg

Sr. Jeanne Bauhs

Sr. Joan Reichelt

Sr. Mary Schneider

Sr. Bonnie Jean Wek

Sr. Valeria Westendorf

Sr. Lucille Welbig

Sr. Mary Ellen Boehnke

Sr. Fanahan Casey

Sr. Martina Kueter

Sr. Ann (Agnes) Foley

Sr. Katherine Scholtz

Sr. Mary Fran Flood

Sr. Agnes Marie Donelan

Sr. Helen Deis

Sr. Margarita Beaner

Sr. Patricia Ann Murphy

Sr. Deanna Butler

Sr. Marie Joseph Schmitz

Sr. Myron Martin

Sr. Margaret Ann Talbott

Sr. Roch Whittaker

Sr. Mary Denis Collins

Sr. Ann Patrick Gannon

Sr. Immaculata Reddy

Sr. Peter Dangel

Sr. Abbey Kennedy

Sr. Annrita Johnson

Sr. Vicky Larson

Sr. Consuelo Covarrubias

Sr. Mary Thomas

Sr. Marie Celeste Sabers

Sr. SaBina Joyce

Sr. Carol Quinn

Yankton
Benedictine Sisters

Sr. Norma Norton

Sr. Joyce Streff

Indexing